S0-AQK-621

Case
Applications
in
Nursing
Leadership
&
Management

Dedication

To my husband, Jay, who always believes in me,
and to the two absolute joys in my life,
my daughters Jilaina and Cali

Case
Applications
in
Nursing
Leadership
&
Management

Karin Polifko-Harris, PhD, RN, CNAA

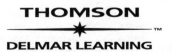

THOMSON

DELMAR LEARNING

Australia, Canada, Mexico, Singapore, Spain, United Kingdom, United States

THOMSON

DELMAR LEARNING

Case Applications in Nursing Leadership & Management

By Karin Polifko-Harris, PhD, RN, CNAA

Vice President, Health Care Business Unit:
William Brottmiller

Editorial Director:
Cathy L. Esperti

Acquisitions Editor:
Matthew Filimonov

Editorial Assistant:
Patricia M. Osborn

Marketing Director:
Jennifer McAvey

Production Editor:
Anne Sherman

RICHARD STOCKTON COLLEGE

3 3005 00708 2472

COPYRIGHT © 2004 by Delmar Learning, a division of Thomson Learning, Inc. Thomson Learning™ is a trademark used herein under license.

Printed in Canada
1 2 3 4 5 XXX 07 06 05 04 03 02

For more information, contact Delmar Learning, 5 Maxwell Drive, Clifton Park, NY 12065 Or find us on the World Wide Web at http://www delmarlearning.com   .

ALL RIGHTS RESERVED. No part of this work covered by the copyright hereon may be reproduced or used in any form or by any means—graphic, electronic, or mechanical, including photocopying, recording, taping, Web distribution or information storage and retrieval systems—without the written permission of the publisher.
For permission to use material from this text or product, contact us by
Tel (800) 730-2214
Fax (800) 730-2215
www.thomsonrights.com

Library of Congress Cataloging-in-Publication Data
Polifko-Harris, Karin, 1958–
  Case applications in nursing leadership & management / by Karin Polifko-Harris.—1st ed.
    p.   ;   cm.
Includes bibliographical references and index.
    ISBN 1-4018-3454-X
  1. Nursing services—Administration—Case studies.
2. Leadership—Case studies.
    [DNLM: 1. Nursing Care—organization & administration—United States—Case Report. 2. Leadership—United States—Case Report. 3. Nurse's Role—United States—Case Report. 4. Patient Care Planning—organization & administration—United States—Case Report. 5. Vocational Guidance—United States—Case Report. WY 105 P767c 2005]   I. Title.
RT89.P646 2005
362.17'3'068—dc22 2003023851

Notice to the Reader

Publisher does not warrant or guarantee any of the products described herein or perform any independent analysis in connection with any of the product information contained herein. Publisher does not assume, and expressly disclaims, any obligation to obtain and include information other than that provided to it by the manufacturer.

The reader is expressly warned to consider and adopt all safety precautions that might be indicated by the activities described herein and to avoid all potential hazards. By following the instructions contained herein, the reader willingly assumes all risks in connection with such instructions.

The publisher makes no representations or warranties of any kind, including but not limited to, the warranties of fitness for particular purpose or merchantability, nor are any such representations implied with respect to the material set forth herein, and the publisher takes no responsibility with respect to such material. The publisher shall not be liable for any special, consequential, or exemplary damages resulting, in whole or part, from the reader's use of, or reliance upon, this material.

RT 89 .P646 2004
53369925
Case applications in nursing
leadership & management

Contents

THE RICHARD STOCKTON COLLEGE
OF NEW JERSEY LIBRARY
POMONA, NEW JERSEY 08240-0195

THE RICHARD STOCKTON COLLEGE
OF NEW JERSEY LIBRARY
POMONA, NEW JERSEY 08240-0195

Margaret M. Anderson RN, EdD, CNAA
Chair, Department of Nursing and Health Professions
Associate Professor of Nursing
Northern Kentucky University
Highland Heights, KY

Pamela P. Cook, RN, MSN, CAN
Assistant Professor of Nursing
Medical College of Georgia
Augusta, GA 30912

Nancy T. Goodman, RNC, MSN
Associate Professor of Nursing
Texas A&M University-Corpus Christi
Corpus Christi, TX

Christy R. Johnson RN, MSN, FNP-C
Associate Professor of Nursing
Gordon College
Barnesville, Georgia

Kathleen Poindexter, RN, MSN
Associate Professor
Ferris State University
Big Rapids, Michigan

Marsha Purtee, RN, MS
Associate Professor of Nursing
Kettering College
Kettering, Ohio

Barbara G. White, RN, MS
Clinical Associate Professor
Arizona State University
Phoenix, AZ

Case Applications in Nursing Leadership & Management is written to assist the nursing student in developing critical thinking, problem-solving, and decision-making abilities in nursing leadership and management situations. This text is designed to be used either in tandem with Patricia Kelly-Heidenthal's *Nursing Leadership & Management* textbook, or to augment another chosen nursing leadership and management text. *Case Applications in Nursing Leadership & Management* contains real-life scenarios that require the student to respond in a logical and rational manner: There are no yes/no responses.

Organization of the Text

Case Applications in Nursing Leadership & Management contains 25 chapters. Topics include management and leadership theories, the changing health care environment, planning for effective nursing care, the delivery and evaluation of care, and professional considerations in the nursing profession.

Each chapter begins with a summary of essential topical concepts, presented as a bulleted list for clear comprehension. The first guided case scenario in a chapter is followed by several case considerations, or questions, that are posed to the student for analysis. In this first case scenario, the student is guided through a case analysis, with the author providing the answers, hence illustrating the depth and level of analysis needed at the manager/leader level. By providing a response, the author is guiding the student through a mentoring process from an experienced leader level. There may be times that the students or faculty may not agree with the author's response; this will present an opportunity for discussion, critical thinking and class debate. Each chapter then contains one to two additional case scenarios with case considerations

and a section entitled Key Points. Key Points are thought-provoking issues for the student to contemplate as they answer the questions presented in the case scenario, again providing a mentoring framework.

A strength of this text is that many of the scenarios have been tested
(and retested!) for years on baccalaureate students enrolled in Leadership and Management courses, providing feedback and revisions long
before they were used in this book. Faculty may also use the case scenarios in the text as assignments or exam questions, tailoring the desired
responses to the individual faculty's particular lecture.

Karin Polifko-Harris is currently the Associate Dean for Academic and Student Affairs at the University of Florida. Dr. Polifko-Harris has held positions in nursing and health care administration, including roles as administrative coordinator for several intensive care units, as director of nursing for critical and medical-surgical care, as clinical specialist in critical care and as vice president for system development and research. Her experience in higher education includes roles as faculty, Chair of the Department of Nursing and Graduate Program Director at a state university in Virginia. She also provides educational and leadership consulting.

Dr. Polifko-Harris earned a bachelor of science in nursing from the University of North Carolina at Charlotte; a master of science in nursing from The University of Pennsylvania where she specialized as an adult nurse practitioner, a post-master's certificate in nursing administration from Villanova University and a PhD in Public Administration from Old Dominion University. She is nationally certified as a Nurse Administrator, Advanced from the American Nurses Credentialing Center.

Professional and community leadership has always been significant for Dr. Polifko-Harris. She has held roles ranging from President of the Society of Critical Care Medicine, Carolinas/Virginia chapter, President of Health Care Administrators of Tidewater (an ACHE chapter), Virginia Nurses Association, State Commissioner on Policies, as well as board memberships on the American Heart Association, the Leukemia Association, the President's Council, International College, the Peninsula Agency on Aging, the Norfolk Senior Center, and serving as a nurse volunteer for the Chesapeake Free Clinic.

Introduction

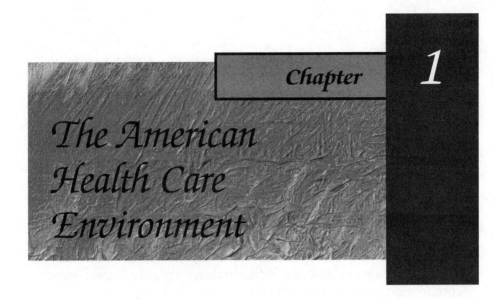

Chapter 1

The American Health Care Environment

Essential Concepts in the American Health Care Environment

America spends more money per capita on health care than any other developed country in the world. Yet, millions of Americans struggle daily with issues of access to as well as with cost and quality of the services that are delivered by the health care systems across the nation.

Many people in the United States believe that everyone is entitled to the same level of heath care and the same services, but that is not always the case. Millions of dollars are spent on the hospital care of premature babies, but ensuring that all pregnant mothers receive prenatal care is simply not a reality in the twenty-first century. In a similar example, advances in technology enable the expertise of health care providers to maintain a person's life after a catastrophic event; however, too little money is spent on the care of chronically ill and aged patients. Many Americans also follow poor health practices, such as smoking, alcohol consumption, overeating, and lack of exercise, leading to unhealthy lifestyles and, eventually, poorer health and outcomes.

3

To strengthen the American health care system, changes continue to affect all levels of health care delivery, ranging from the primary care system of preventative care to the secondary, acute hospitalization phase to tertiary rehabilitative services. The reimbursement system continues to refine itself as more acute care systems apply clinical pathways and clinical informatics to improve outcomes and measures of quality. In turn, issues of recruitment and retention are constantly being reviewed and revised to ensure a competent workforce at all levels while monitoring the supply and demand of both professionals and allied health workers.

Organization of Health Care in America

- Health care in the United States was designed within a political framework that emphasized individualism, equality of processes, competition, and the Protestant work ethic.
- Health care is managed by a variety of agencies, including federal, state, local, and private organizations.
- Health care delivery is not equally accessed by all Americans.
- Primary health care services are predominately preventative in nature, with a secondary focus on the acute phase of illness. Tertiary services are those with a rehabilitative or restorative concentration.
- Title XVIII of the Social Security Act Amendments formulated Medicare, with Medicaid arising out of Title XIX. Simply stated, Medicare provides health care services to patients who are older than 65 years and to patients who are the disabled, while Medicaid is for those who are the medically indigent, regardless of age (http://www.medicare.gov).
- Historically, health care services were reimbursed under a fee-for-service program, in which all charges were reimbursed to the provider and hospitals, regardless of the actual costs. This type of reimbursement system encouraged a higher number of patient services, whether these services were medically indicated or not.
- Because of cost-containment measures when health care services and providers' charges continued to grow, in 1982 Congress passed the Tax Equity and Fiscal Responsibility Act (TEFRA), which spawned the prospective payment system (PPS) (Jonas & Kovner, 1992).

Movement Toward Population-Based Health Care and Disease Management

- Rather than focusing on the health care needs of an individual, population-based health care involves studying the effects of health, illness, and death on a group of people.

- With population-based health care, the focus is on keeping the population healthy (rather than on caring for a population once it becomes ill) and on the various diseases and causative factors. The United States, in its efforts to increase prevention of disease and illnesses, needs to continually redirect resources toward strengthening health, including lifestyle choices; influences on work, home, and school; and environmental influences on the community.
- *Healthy People 2010* (http://www.healthypeople.gov), issued by the United States Department of Health and Human Services, assists communities in prioritizing health achievement and maintenance initiatives, such as disease prevention, smoking cessation, early prenatal care, and immunizations for children.

Health Care Variation and Evidence-Based Practice

- Many causative factors (variations) influence patient care outcomes (results).
- Evidence-based practice means applying practice guidelines to producing the best possible clinical outcomes for the patient. For example, when a facility develops a clinical guideline for the best practice of caring for patients after a hip replacement, it will examine the evidence of best practice by all the physicians who perform this type of surgery, looking for low infection rates, early ambulation, and early discharge.
- Best practice guidelines are a compilation of patient outcomes that result in the optimal care. One example is that to effectively discharge a patient receiving a hip replacement on the fourth postoperative day, ambulation may begin the first rather than on the second postoperative day.

Current Trends and Forces Influencing Health Care Delivery

- The Health Insurance Portability and Accountability Act (HIPAA) was designed in 1996 to provide patients with privacy, security, and confidentiality as their information is transmitted during the billing, claims processing, and reimbursement phases. As of April 2003, this act is fully in place in all health care agencies (Kumekawa, 2001).
- Information about the quality of physicians, health care systems, and health care plans is increasingly available, not only in print but also on the Internet. One indirect potential goal in making much of this information available is to encourage the public to take the initiative in finding out the quality of services provided.

Table 1-1   Pew Health Professions Competencies

1. Embrace a personal ethic of social responsibility and service.
2. Exhibit ethical behavior in all professional activities.
3. Provide evidence-based, clinically competent care.
4. Incorporate the multiple determinants of health in clinical care.
5. Apply knowledge of the new sciences.
6. Demonstrate critical thinking, reflection, and problem-solving skills.
7. Understand the role of primary care.
8. Rigorously practice preventive health care.
9. Integrate population-based care and services into practices.
10. Improve access to health care for those with unmet health needs.
11. Practice relationship-centered care with individuals and families.
12. Provide culturally sensitive care to a diverse society.
13. Partner with communities in health care decisions.
14. Use communication and information technology effectively and appropriately.
15. Work in interdisciplinary teams.
16. Ensure care that balances individual, professional, system, and societal needs.
17. Practice leadership.
18. Take responsibility for quality of care and health outcomes at all levels.
19. Contribute to continuous improvement of the health care system.
20. Advocate for public policy that promotes and protects the health of the public.
21. Continue to learn and help others learn.

Reprinted from O'Neil & the Pew Professions Commission (1998); with permission.

If the information is public, then hopefully, a sustained effort will be made to increase and maintain quality services with quality outcomes.
- The Pew Health Professions Commission Report (O'Neil & the Pew Professions Commission, 1998) wrote 21 competencies for nursing, medical, and other health care providers to strive to achieve for the twenty-first century (Table 1-1).
- Additional changes that affect health care delivery include the continuation of managed care influences (e.g., capitation), clinical pathways, new technology, a changing workforce, changing demographics in the United States, clinical informatics, social morbidity, and changing societal values.
- Nursing roles continue to evolve and expand as the need for interdisciplinary skills and leadership continue to grow.

CASE SCENARIOS

Guided Case Scenario 1-1

You are working the evening shift in the Emergency Department when you notice Mrs. Pittman in the triage area. Mrs. Pittman is known by all the staff members in the emergency room, because she is there almost once a week with similar complaints of dizziness, high blood pressure, and side effects of alcohol consumption.

Mrs. Pittman does not have family members, or at least she does not admit to having any family in town. You know that her diagnoses include type 1 diabetes, obesity, hypertension, and chronic alcoholism. She is unemployed and receives government assistance. You are unsure of her living conditions.

Tonight, she presents with shortness of breath and extreme thirst. After examining Mrs. Pittman, a new physician working in the department asks that you "take care of Mrs. Pittman so that she doesn't come back into the Emergency Department so frequently with the same problems."

Case Considerations

1. Where do you begin with Mrs. Pittman? Her case seems almost overwhelming to you.
2. What are some of the variables that can be addressed if concepts of population-based care are applied?
3. How can Mrs. Pittman best be assisted in decreasing her recidivism in the Emergency Department?
4. Identify several social and medical resources to assist Mrs. Pittman.

Case Analysis

1. Where do you begin with Mrs. Pittman? Her case seems almost overwhelming to you.

   Mrs. Pittman's case may seem almost overwhelming, but this situation is not unusual or unknown to many emergency departments across the country. Obviously, she has several chronic diseases, has limited resources in dealing with her chronic health problems, and turns to the Emergency Department as her primary source of medical care.

In working with Mrs. Pittman, it is important to look first at this case in the broad sense rather than to look at only one or two details. Look at the big picture of Mrs. Pittman to prioritize her needs, possibly even applying Maslow's Hierarchy of Needs. If you look only at a specific health issue (e.g., her type 1 diabetes), then you are not taking into account many of the influencing factors that affect her overall health condition. At this point, it is helpful to ask other resources (e.g., staff) who may be better qualified to begin working with Mrs. Pittman in hopes of decreasing her frequent visits to the emergency department.

2. What are some of the variables that can be addressed if concepts of population-based care are applied?

    To be effective with Mrs. Pittman, the most important step is to contact those who know not only the health care system but also the resources available in the local community. As an emergency room nurse, you may be in the position to initiate a referral, perhaps a key provider; however, because of your scope of practice, you cannot take on Mrs. Pittman's case by yourself. Most emergency departments have either a case manager or a social worker who is assigned exclusively to this area to take care of clients such as Mrs. Pittman. It is in the best interests of the institution, the health care providers, and most of all, Mrs. Pittman to have her chronic diseases more effectively controlled so that she is not visiting the Emergency Department on a weekly basis. With population-based care, prevention rather than treatment of the illness is the goal. It appears that Mrs. Pittman has several variables to consider, including her medical illnesses of diabetes, hypertension, and chronic alcoholism, along with her social issues of unemployment and lack of social and family support systems.

    A significant issue to understand is that this client may not have the resources that others have when becoming ill. To whom does she turn when problems of shelter, food, money, and health arise? What are the social and medical resources Mrs. Pittman needs, and does she even have access to those services? Does she have the financial resources? Finally, does she have the necessary knowledge to maintain her health and to understand her diseases?

3. How can Mrs. Pittman best be assisted in decreasing her recidivism in the Emergency Department?

The first step is to contact someone either in the Case Management Department or in the Social Services Department for assistance with Mrs. Pittman's case. This is not a case that you, as an emergency room nurse, can handle by yourself.

4. Identify several social and medical resources to assist Mrs. Pittman.

Once you have contacted the Social Services or Case Management Department, you can look to see what other personnel resources may be available in your institution. The social worker or case manager can often coordinate the care, especially when the patient is seen frequently for the same diagnoses. Social workers have community connections with various social service and governmental agencies that can greatly assist clients with issues of access, housing, medical, and funding resources.

Most facilities also have pastoral care, which is helpful in offering solace and compassion to someone who feels alone. There may be a patient educator who can be brought in to ensure that Mrs. Pittman has at least a basic understanding of her chronic diseases, and there may be a diabetes educator who can offer more in-depth information. The essential point to remember is that Mrs. Pittman is the type of patient with care needs that are complex and require coordination from several sources. Although she seeks medical care for her health issues, other issues, such as adequate food, shelter, and money, may be the underlying reasons for her noncompliance in taking care of her health.

Case Scenario 1-2

One of your patient's wives, Mrs. Agape, comes up to you one afternoon at work. She says she is confused over some of the billing from her husband's last hospitalization but does not want to bother her husband's doctor with questions. She says that her insurer has changed the rules so many times she does not even know many of the terms they use and what she can expect from them. She asks you what has happened to hospitals in the last few years to make them dramatically change how they do business.

Case Considerations

1. What would you first say to Mrs. Agape about managed care? What exactly does this term mean to her as a recipient of health care in the United States?

2. If a patient has problems with their bill from the hospital, how would you advise them?
3. Are there any other resources you can offer to Mrs. Agape to help her better understand the current health care environment in general and her insurance issues in particular?
4. Describe the significant changes in the business of hospital care during the last decade and what drove those changes.

Case Analysis

The health care environment has changed dramatically since the mid-1980s not only for patients but also for health care providers and institutions. Answering Mrs. Agape's questions about managed care both quickly and succinctly is not an easy task, so you need to prioritize what you believe are the critical points that will help her to gain a basic understanding. The significant question for Mrs. Agape, however, is not necessarily about managed care but, rather, about her bill from the hospital.

■ KEY POINTS

1. In reviewing the priority question of billing, to whom would you refer Mrs. Agape? Who would the best resources be to review her bill? Why is this a priority with Mrs. Agape?
2. The health care environment has significantly changed during the last two decades. What are some key points to make with any patient or their family so that they can begin to understand the issues? What are some of the newer changes in health care?
3. How much information should you share about the quality of the physician's care? Where would you guide a family seeking this information?
4. Are there any other resources within the hospital setting to whom you can refer Mrs. Agape so that she can better understand the managed care environment? Are there any outside resources?

References

Jonas, S., & Kovner, A. R. (2002). *Health care delivery in the United States* (7th ed.) New York: Springer Publishing.

Kumekawa, J. K. (2001). Health information privacy protection: Crisis or common sense? *Online Journal of Issues in Nursing*, 6 (3), 14.

O'Neil, E. H., & the Pew Professions Committee. (1998). *Recreating health professional practice for a new century.* San Francisco: Pew Health Professions Commissions.

Suggested Readings

Bellack, J. P., & O'Neil, E. H. (2000). Recreating nursing practice for a new century: Recommendations and implications of the Pew Health Professions Commission's final report. *Nursing and Health Care Perspectives, 21* (1), 1–14.

Byers, S. A. (1997). *The executive nurse—Leadership for new health transitions.* Clifton Park, NY: Delmar Learning.

Fos, P. J., & Fine, D. J. (2000). *Designing health care for populations.* San Francisco: Jossey-Bass.

Joint Commission on Accreditation of Healthcare Organizations. (2001). *Manual for hospitals.* Chicago: Joint Commission on Accreditation of Healthcare Organizations.

Kohn, L., Corrigan, J., & Donaldson, M. (Eds.). (2001). *Crossing the quality chasm: A new health system for the 21st century.* Washington, D.C.: Committee on Quality of Care in America, Institute of Medicine, National Academy Press.

Kongstvedt, P. (2002). *Managed care: What it is and how it works.* Gaithersburg, MD: Aspen Publishers.

Lang, N. M. (1999). Discipline approaches to evidence-based practice: A view from nursing. *Joint Commission Journal on Quality Improvement, 25* (10), 539–544.

McCormick, K. A., Cummings, M. A., & Kovner, C. (1997). The role of the Agency for Health Care Policy and Research in improving outcomes of care. *Nursing Clinics of North America, 32* (3), 5.

Morrissey, J. (2001, January 1). Slow down: HIPPA ahead. *Modern Healthcare, 30.*

U.S. Department of Health and Human Services. (2000). *Healthy people 2010.* Washington, D.C.: U.S. Government Printing Office.

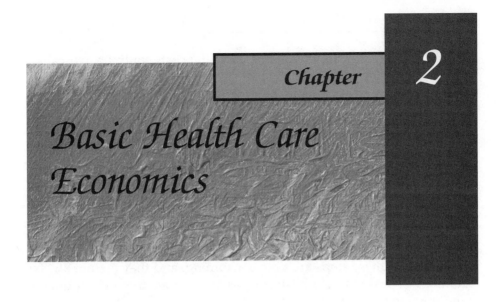

Chapter 2

Basic Health Care Economics

Essential Concepts of Health Care Economics

The health care financing system has undergone significant changes since the early 1980s, when most payments were made to physicians and hospitals in a retrospective manner, regardless of the actual costs to perform the service or what the provider charged. The advent of managed care has changed the reimbursement system to that of a prospective payment system (PPS), with monetary parameters in place that often limit spending and reimbursement. Payment for health care services in the United States is increasingly coming from a blend of private and public entities. Unlike other developed countries, the United States does not pay entirely for health care services out of public funds; instead, it relies heavily on employer and private citizen contributions.

Key words in the managed care triad are *cost, access,* and *quality.* This chapter deals with many of the cost issues affecting health care delivery and examines health care as a business. By focusing more on the business aspect of health care delivery, providers and consumers alike show a concern with the rising costs, not only for insurance purposes but also for the purchasing of services, such as pharmaceuticals, disposable materials, and other care modalities. Hospital costs continue to escalate, with expenses for diagnostic, therapeutic, and information technology often surpassing the personnel budget. Many facilities submit a Certificate of Need (CON) to their states when considering the purchase of expensive technology in an effort not to duplicate services already in place.

Nursing continues to be a labor-intensive budget item in all acute care facilities. Several steps can be taken to identify nursing costs. These steps include applying a patient classification system, determining the relative value units of nursing care delivered, and reviewing the staffing mix to ensure that more expensive registered nurses are not performing less technical skills, which can be delegated more effectively to unlicensed personnel. All these steps are time-consuming, and they are not always embraced by hospital administrators as an accurate method for quantifying nursing costs in a facility.

Health Care as a Business

- Economics is the study of allocating scarce resources in an appropriate manner.
- Although health care is a business, many consumers view health care differently from the traditional economics model: Many do not "price shop" to ensure the optimal price (the best value for cost) or examine the issue of payment options available to the consumer.
- Americans hold a generalized viewpoint that health care is to be offered to all, regardless of the cost, access, or quality of care, and that the provider rather than the consumer should determine the actual need for health care services.

Cost as a Consideration in Health Care Options

- Most people hold a right to health care at a reasonable cost as an inherent American value. A reasonable cost is defined as the usual and customary fees (charges) depending on the section of the country: Different areas of a state may charge more or less for the same procedure.
- Health care reform began with the onset of managed care in an effort to control the costs of Medicare and Medicaid programs.
- Managed care is "a system of health care delivery that tries to control the cost of health care services while regulating access to those services and maintaining or improving their quality" (Kongstvedt, 2002, p. 285).
- Key words in the managed care triad are *cost*, *access*, and *quality*.

- Various models of managed care health care systems exist, including the health maintenance organization (HMO) and the preferred provider organization (PPO).
- Socialized medicine provides universal access to health care, from preventive care to acute care, for an entire community of people.

Issues Influencing Basic Health Care Economics

- Complex and expensive technologies (e.g., diagnostic and therapeutic technologies), computerization, and competition for the newest services all contribute to the increase in health care costs.
- Health care providers, especially in the nursing and allied health professionals, are in great demand because the number of students entering these professions has decreased. When a decrease occurs in supply, a subsequent increase often occurs in demand.
- Health care has taken on a more business-like focus, often coming in conflict with an agency's mission to provide care regardless of a patient's ability to pay. Profits are more important than ever, with the health care industry looking more closely at the system's revenues and costs.
- Fundamental costs to health care include direct costs, indirect costs, fixed costs, and variable costs. Increasingly, first-line managers are responsible for their department's budget plan.
- Health care systems are undertaking a rationing approach to providing health care services, resulting in numerous potential ramifications and ethical debates.
- Historically, nursing is one area of acute care services in which it has been difficult to determine direct costs. Several methods, including the Patient Classification System and the Relative Value Unit, along with measures of quality practice, have assisted some nursing systems in identifying their contributions to the larger health care system.

CASE SCENARIOS

Guided Case Scenario 2-1

In a scene familiar to many during the last few years, the Chief Nursing Officer (CNO) calls a meeting of the 10 nurse managers at St. Monica's Hospital to discuss issues relating to escalating costs, nursing care delivery, and the quality of care provided. The CNO arrives at the meeting with nothing more than a blank tablet. She begins the discussion by stating that the fiscal resources at St. Monica's are getting tighter and that, like the three other administrators, she has been asked to look at both revenues and costs to ascertain if there are ways to curtail expenses. You were just hired less than a month ago as the new nurse manager of a 50-bed medical surgical unit, and although you manage the largest unit, you also have the most vacancies, have the largest variety of physicians, and often take overflow from the other units. Your CNO begins the discussion with you and asks where you believe costs can be cut.

Case Considerations

1. Where do you begin, especially when you have just started your new position and have not yet had time to meet all the physicians?
2. What are some critical pieces of information you will need before you can even begin to offer suggestions to your CNO?
3. What information can your staff provide to you, especially those who have been employed for a significant length of time?
4. Who is responsible for measuring the quality of care?

Case Analysis

1. Where do you begin, especially when you have just started your new position and have not yet had time to meet all the physicians?

   Before you offer suggestions, you may want to spend valuable time observing your staff, the physicians, and the patients. First, how efficient is your staff in accomplishing daily tasks and assignments? Are they able to begin and complete an assignment with minimal effort, or do they spend a fair amount of time searching for and replacing items that are missing, broken, or perhaps, even hidden somewhere? Are medications easily available, or do runners constantly need to go between the unit and the pharmacy for even basic medications?

   Another area to look at is the staffing mix. What is your percentage of registered nurses (RNs)? Of licensed practical nurses (LPNs)? Of unlicensed assistive personnel (UAPs)? How well do the RNs supervise and work with the staff? Is the secretarial support sufficient for the unit? Is someone primarily in charge of customer satisfaction? How satisfied is the staff with their work environment? With the hospital leadership? If they are not entirely satisfied, is this situation leading to a high turnover rate?

What type of interaction occurs between the physicians and nurses? Is it a respectful relationship, or is it fraught with tension? Do you see certain physicians more often than others? What type of quality care do they deliver? Are they responsive to patient complications? Are there risk management issues with numerous incidences?

What type of patients does your unit have, and what is the average acuity level? Are they primarily patients who are ambulatory, or are they bedridden and requiring many hours of nursing care? Do they have families, or are many single? What is the age range? What are the diagnoses? Are there any other system issues that may have been overlooked?

2. What are some critical pieces of information that you will need before you can even begin to offer suggestions to your CNO?

Several important pieces of information can assist you as you prepare your presentation to the CNO. First, you should know what percentage of your patients are Medicare, Medicaid, private insurance, or self-pay by knowing the reimbursement rates for each of these patient sources. By knowing the primary insurers, you can build a picture of your unit's patient population.

Second, it is helpful to know how many employees your unit would have if fully staffed and which positions are RNs, LPNs, and UAPs. How many vacancies are there? In what category do the vacancies occur? Are there an abundance of per diem, agency, or travelers on the unit, resulting in higher personnel costs? Is the amount of overtime, sick, and vacation time abused?

Third, who are the physicians with the highest numbers of patients admitted to your unit? What is their relationship with the professional staff? With what type of patients do they work? Are the patients surgical or medical?

Lastly, what type of overflow patients are admitted to your unit? Under what circumstances are they admitted? Are they appropriately admitted, or are they patients who other units do not necessarily want to take care of, either because of complexity or chronicity?

3. What information can your staff provide to you, especially those who have been employed for a significant length of time?

One issue in this area is a high vacancy rate. Staff who have
been employed for any length of time can assist you, as a new
manager, in seeing some of the underlying tensions and issues
relating to turnover. What is the general perception of the
staff? How satisfied are they professionally? How do the staff
feel about their pay? About their benefit package? Do the staff
feel appreciated and acknowledged? All these issues are not
readily found listed in staffing grids or discussed at staff meetings but, instead, can be explored by asking staff about them,
either on a one-by-one basis or through a questionnaire. These
factors are critical when reviewing retention concerns.

4. Who is responsible for measuring the quality of care?

Quality care is the responsibility of everyone who provides
any level of care to a patient, regardless of his or her status or
job position. If only one or two people have formal, designated
responsibility for maintaining quality care, then you, as the
new manager, may have a more difficult time getting all staff
members to acknowledge their responsibility to the patient.

Case Scenario 2-2

Just about every day, one can hear a physician, nurse, or hospital
administrator discussing how health care has turned into a business.
A newly graduated RN just started on your unit, and she states that
she went into the nursing profession to help take care of people who
are not able to help themselves. She does not appear to be quite sure
what to make of all these conversations. She comes into the break
room and joins some of the more experienced staff, including you.
She says that she wants help in understanding why health care has
become more of a business during the last few decades, because the
reality of health care is not what she had envisioned.

Case Considerations

1. What would you begin to tell this new graduate?
2. What are some key points to make to her about the business of
   health care today?
3. What are some of the advantages and disadvantages to having
   a business focus in health care?

Case Analysis

You do not want to be negative about the fact that health care
has changed over the last several decades and taken on a more

business-like approach. You do, however, need to be realistic about the current health care environment and the expectations that all nursing staff must fulfill to provide effective and efficient care.

■ KEY POINTS

1. Nursing is a high-touch profession that has, as its base, a caring attitude toward another human being. No matter how much the business components may influence health care delivery, it is critical to keep your perspective about nursing care. How would you reassure the new graduate that although health care is a business, nursing is still—and will always be—a profession that works intimately with its patients?
2. Why has health care evolved into more of a business model? What are some of the factors contributing to this change?
3. What are some of the accepted values placed on health care delivery by the American public?
4. What are some of the fundamental costs in health care? What costs have increased disproportionately over the last few years?

Reference

Kongstvedt, P. (2002). *Managed care: What it is and how it works.* Gaithersburg, MD: Aspen Publishers.

Suggested Readings

Antia, N. A. (2001). Health economics or the economics of health? *Journal of Health Management,* 3 (2), 159–165.

Finkler, S. A. (2001). *Budgeting concepts for nurse managers* (3rd ed.). Philadelphia: W. B. Saunders.

Finkler, S. A., & Kovner, C. T. (2000). *Financial management for nurse managers and nurse executives* (2nd ed.). Philadelphia: W. B. Saunders.

Griggith, J. (1999). *The well-managed health care organization.* Chicago: Health Administration Press.

Jonas, S., & Kovner, A. R. (2002). *Health care delivery in the United States* (7th ed.). New York: Springer Publishing.

Kongstvedt, P. (2001). *Essentials in managed care* (4th ed.). Gaithersburg, MD: Aspen Publishers.

Kramer, M., & Schmalenberg, C. (2002). Essentials of magnetism. In: M. McClure & A. S. Hinshaw (Eds.), *Magnet hospitals revisited: Attraction and retention of professional nurses.* Kansas City, MO: American Academy of Nurses.

Meisenheimer, C. G. (1997). *Improving quality.* Gaithersburg, MD: Aspen Publishers.

O'Dowd, A. (2002). Setting the new agenda. *Nursing Times, 98* (49), 22-25.

Quintero, J. R. (2003). Progressive care. Achieve cost benefits with innovative care management. *Critical Care Nurse, 23* (2), 109–113.

Rosenblatt, R. A. (2002). Health politics: Here we go again. *Aging Today, 23* (3), 1–2.

Scott, J., Sochalski, J., & Aiken, L. (1999). Review of magnet hospital research. *Journal of Nursing Administration, 29,* 9–19.

Shui, L., & Singh, D. A. (1998). *Delivering health care in America.* Gaithersburg, MD: Aspen Publishers.

Stewart, K. (2003). Seven ways to help your hospital stay in business: Your inpatient decisions can make or break your local hospital. *Family Practice Management, 10* (5), 27–30, 78–79.

Sultz, H. A., & Young, K. M. (1999). *Health care USA* (2nd ed.). Gaithersburg, MD: Aspen Publishers.

Wolper, L. (1999). *Health care administration planning, implementing and managing organized delivery systems* (3rd ed.). Gaithersburg, MD: Aspen Publishers.

A New Health Care Model

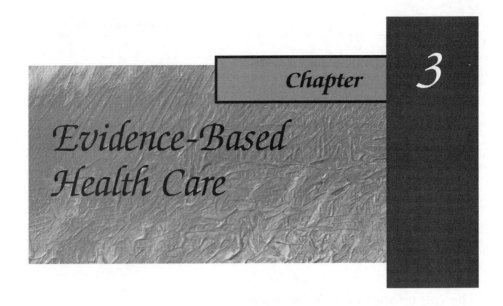

Chapter *3*

Evidence-Based Health Care

Essential Concepts of Evidence-Based Health Care

Nurses have been providing evidence-based care (EBC) since the profession began. A need has always existed for nurses to provide competent nursing care, which is based on current research and facts, with the goal to evaluate the care's effectiveness toward positive patient outcomes. Historically, the profession has relied on basic research methods to illustrate the effects of nursing care, newer technologies and methods that lend themselves to even more sophisticated results.

Evidence-based health care is appropriately applied to all providers who want to make accurate decisions about patient care based on the scientific method of inquiry. This process of scientific inquiry includes collecting, analyzing, interpreting, and critiquing the results obtained from a certain patient population as well as comparing these results to those found in the literature and other sources to ensure that best practices are, indeed, maintained.

History of Evidence-Based Care

- The term *evidence-based care* was first identified at McMaster Medical School in Canada during 1980s as an attempt to integrate a practitioner's care with systematic, research-based, clinical evidence (Rosen & Donald, 1995).
- EBC is multidisciplinary in nature and includes all types of clinical health care providers, such as nurses and physicians, who need to work collaboratively to ensure the best outcomes for their patients.
- Journals and other sources provide media for review of clinical data that can then be interpreted and analyzed for best practice techniques.

The Importance of Evidence-Based Care

- The underlying assumption of EBC is that its goal for nursing, medicine, and allied health care practitioners is to provide optimal care using the most current scientific knowledge available, resulting in optimal patient results or outcomes.
- EBC should be viewed as providing the highest standard of care for the patient.

Issues that Support an Evidence-Based Care Model

- Nurses as well as physicians need to demonstrate that the outcomes of health care not only benefit the patient but also are cost-effective, are of quality, and are medically effective and safe.
- The managed care environment has challenged health care institutions to move patients through the system in a more efficient and effective manner and, often, to look at other institutions for their best practice ideas in an effort to decrease costs.
- Nurses can be strong advocates of EBC, because they deal with the patient and his or her family 24 hours a day and are best positioned to see any variance in the expected or desired outcomes.
- The Joint Commission on Accreditation of Healthcare Organizations (JCAHO; http://www.jcaho.org) has recently put into place requirements for institutions to establish EBC standards of care.
- In 1997, the Agency for Healthcare Research and Quality (AHRQ; http://www.ahrq.com) began publishing data for 12 evidence-based practice centers. One goal of the AHRQ is to assist health care providers and institutions to improve the quality and effectiveness and to determine the necessity of certain aspects of patient care.

CASE SCENARIOS

Guided Case Scenario 3-1

A new surgeon, Dr. Reed, who recently completed her residency, joins the staff at Merry Marker Hospital. Dr. Reed's specialty is orthopedics, and it appears that the majority of her surgeries are hip replacements. As the nurse manager of the surgical floor, you notice that Dr. Reed's outcomes are quite different from the rest of the orthopedic physicians, all of whom have been practicing at Merry Marker for many years. Dr. Reed's patients undergoing hip replacement are out of bed the day after surgery, are ambulating that evening, and are often discharged home by the fourth day. The other patients do not get fully out of bed until about the third day, and they seem to have more complications that require not only more resources but also delays in discharge. You realize that Dr. Reed's patients appear to have significantly better outcomes than the other patients on your unit undergoing the same procedure.

Case Considerations

1. How would one validate the outcomes of Dr. Reed's patients?
2. What care outcomes should be reviewed and why?
3. How should one organize the validation process?
4. Who should be involved in this research?
5. What value does this research have? Who else in the hospital would be interested in the results?
6. How would other physicians become involved?

Case Analysis

1. How would one validate the outcomes of Dr. Reed's patients?

   If general observation is telling you that a difference exists in the outcomes between Dr. Reed and the other physicians on the staff, then you have already begun the research process into determining patient care outcomes using EBC. If you have not done a project such as this before, you may want to seek guidance from someone in the organization who has or from someone who is responsible for the patient care outcomes in the institution, such as from the Quality Management Department.

2. What care outcomes should be reviewed and why?

The most important outcomes are those that are related to patient care. You could begin with basic outcomes that are easily measured and are usually kept by someone in the organization. Lengths of stay and infection rates for postoperative hip replacements are two easy data points that are always collected and reviewed, regardless of the institution. One can also look at the costs involved per case, the day of first ambulation, or any number of physician-related outcomes.

3. How should one organize the validation process?

In organizing the research project, you begin with planning to collect the appropriate data. Then, you move on to collecting the actual data, analyzing the data, summarizing the findings, and applying the findings to the current situation.

It is important to spend adequate time in the beginning to plan what type of data will be collected. The wrong type of data will yield results that may not be meaningful or that may be too complex to reach a true analysis. When collecting the data, you have to ensure that the collection is unbiased (not favoring one physician over another). Drawing conclusions and making recommendations are much easier using objective data versus subjective data; however, both types of data have their place in the research process.

4. Who should be involved in this research?

Depending on your skill level and on that of the staff, many people in an acute care facility can assist in the process of data gathering, interpretation, and evaluation. If you are looking at medical outcomes, it is critical to gain the early support of the physicians, perhaps through the Unit Medical Director or the Chief of Staff. The Chief Nursing Officer, as well as his or her designee, should also be included among those who need to be aware of this project.

Within the organization, other resources may be able to assist you, because they are already collecting certain data. Perhaps the Quality Improvement Director, the Case Manager assigned to your unit, the Risk Manager, and anyone else responsible for outcome management in the facility could assist. Another possibility is to engage nursing faculty from a local college to assist you in setting up your study and ensuring that you are reviewing the data correctly.

5. What value does this research have? Who else in the hospital would be interested in the results?

It is always a goal of any health care institution or provider to give the best care possible. The overarching purpose of EBC is to do just that: using data, finding the best practices, and encouraging others to use these practices.

Increasing the quality of any service can only improve an institution's reputation, assure that patients are receiving the best care possible, and attract the best nurses, physicians, and other health care providers as well as ancillary services. Others who would be interested in your results would be stakeholders both inside and outside the institution. Inside stakeholders would be other physicians, administrators, board members, patients, and their families. Outside stakeholders would be the community, the newspapers and other media, competing hospitals, physicians, and potential patients and their families.

6. How would other physicians become involved?

This may be a difficult step unless you have a physician "champion," someone the other physicians respect and who demonstrates best practices. It is also helpful early in the project to secure the assistance of the Unit Medical Director and the hospital's Medical Chief of Staff.

Case Scenario 3-2

You have decided to implement the research project discussed in Case Scenario 3-1. You present the information at the monthly staff meeting, when one of the registered nurses says, "It all sounds so foreign to me. What is this research all about?" Wanting to take advantage of this question, you begin to immediately plan how to best in-service your staff on the research process, ensuring that they understand some of the basic terminology and processes.

Case Considerations

1. How would you plan your in-service for your staff?
2. What research terms should be familiar to them?
3. How can they assist in the research process?

Case Analysis

This is a wonderful opportunity for staff to participate in the EBC process. By taking the time up-front to help them understand the basic principles of the research process, you lay the groundwork not only for future EBC processes but also for generalized performance improvement activities. Obtaining buy-in early during the process almost assures that staff will become more involved than if they are simply told they need to participate in a process they know little about, especially when the benefits of the research can be made clear.

■ *KEY POINTS*

1. The research process is essentially what nurses do on a daily basis because of the nursing process itself. The nursing process consists of assessment, nursing diagnosis, planning, implementing, and evaluating care.
2. It is valuable that the staff understand some of the terminology of the research process, but why one performs research and its benefits to the patient should be the emphasis.
3. It is important that the staff understand the value of providing EBC for the patient.
4. It would be helpful to see if others in the organization may be able to assist in preparing your in-service. Does the hospital have an Education Department? Are there Clinical Nurse Specialists in the organization who can be used as resources?

Reference

Rosen, W, & Donald, A. (1995). Evidence based medicine: An approach to clinical problem-solving. *British Medical Journal, 310,* 1122–1125.

Suggested Readings

Anderson, C. A. (1998). Does evidence-based practice equal quality nursing care? *Nursing Outlook, 46,* 257–258.

French, P. (1999). The development of evidence-based nursing. *Journal of Advanced Nursing, 29* (1), 72–78.

Goode, C. J. (2000). What constitutes the "evidence" in evidence-based practice? *Applied Nursing Research, 13,* 222–225.

Griggith, J. (1999). *The well-managed health care organization.* Chicago: Health Administration Press.

Haynes, E. (2000). Research as a key to promoting and sustaining innovative practice. *Nursing Clinics of North America, 35,* 453–463.

Jonas, S., & Kovner, A. R. (2002). *Health care delivery in the United States* (7th ed.). New York: Springer Publishing.

Kongstvedt, P. (2001). *Essentials in managed care* (4th ed.). Gaithersburg, MD: Aspen Publishers.

Kongstvedt, P. (2002). *Managed care: What it is and how it works.* Gaithersburg, MD: Aspen Publishers.

Lang, N. M. (1999). Discipline-based approaches to evidence-based practice: A view from nursing. *Joint Commission on Quality Improvement, 25,* 539–544.

Meisenheimer, C. G. (1997). *Improving quality.* Gaithersburg, MD: Aspen Publishers.

Pravikoff, D. S., Pierce, S., & Tanner, A. (2003). Nursing resources. Are nurses ready for evidence-based practice? *American Journal of Nursing, 103* (5), 95–96.

Rambur, B. (1999). Fostering evidence-based practice in nursing education. *Journal of Professional Nursing, 15,* 270–274.

Shui, L., & Singh, D. A. (1998). *Delivering health care in America.* Gaithersburg, MD: Aspen Publishers.

Sultz, H. A., & Young, K. M. (1999). *Health care USA* (2nd ed.). Gaithersburg, MD: Aspen Publishers.

Wolper, L. (1999). *Health care administration planning, implementing and managing organized delivery systems* (3rd ed.). Gaithersburg, MD: Aspen Publishers.

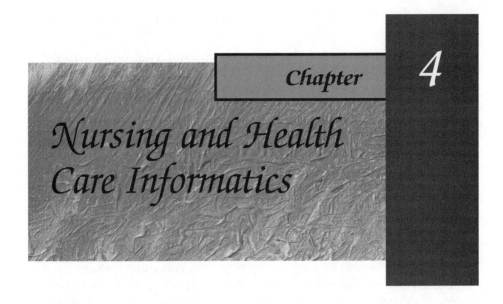

Chapter 4

Nursing and Health Care Informatics

Essential Concepts in Health Care Informatics

Computers define almost everything that we do in health care today. Patients acquire much of their medical education via the Internet. We obtain laboratory values from a computer. We chart patient results in a computer. Physicians can enter orders directly into a computer, and we can evaluate outcomes of patient care using a computer.

Informatics is simply the translation of clinical information into data that are easily read and understood, using technology such as computerization. Clinical information systems include order entry and reporting, documentation, and retrieval of information. Nurses who specialize in informatics often have advanced training in the field and may even have graduate preparation.

Defining the Profession of Nursing Informatics

- Informatics is the study of computer science and information science, including aspects of health care technology ranging from basic to application.

- The definition of nursing informatics from the American Nurses Association (ANA; 1994) includes information that is directly applicable to the work of nursing as well as clinical information management, integration of knowledge from other disciplines, and application of informatics to nursing practice.
- Clinical information systems have changed the ways that hospitals process all patient-related matters, from admissions to discharges to identifying and applying indicators of quality care and outcomes. Informatics has a dramatic impact on all aspects of patient care delivery.
- Computerized patient care records have eliminated the majority of the paper that is contained in a record. Now, the entire client's medical and health history is contained via computerization.
- Security is a significant focus within a computerized patient care record system as well as in a clinical informatics system. Confidentiality is of paramount importance, and measures are put in place to safeguard the information and to control who has access to the data while also adhering to regulations, standards, and applicable laws.
- Three terms specific to the security of a computerized system include *privacy, confidentiality,* and *security.* Privacy is the right of the individual to prevent their personal information from being discussed by unwanted persons. Confidentiality limits the disclosure of personal information. Security ensures that access to information is controlled and protected.

Defining a Nursing Specialty and Informatics as a Nursing Specialty

- In defining a nursing specialty, several components need to be present: specialty practice, a program of research to further the specialty, a recognized organization that represents the specialty, a methodology for credentialing nurses in the specialty, and available educational programs.
- Nursing informatics meets the requirements of a nursing specialty.
- Numerous organizations exist that focus on the field of nursing informatics, including special interest groups in the ANA and the National League for Nursing as well as those outside the nursing profession.
- Increasingly more higher education programs are teaching both undergraduate and graduate students about nursing informatics and its application to patient care delivery.

- Several professional journals include information about nursing informatics, including the *Journal of the American Medical Informatics Association and Computers in Nursing.*
- The American Nurses Credentialing Center (http://www. nursingworld.org) offers a certification examination in nursing informatics.
- Informatics nurses can choose a variety of settings in which to practice, including both acute care and outpatient care centers, insurance companies, managed care organizations, and software-development companies.

Trends in Ubiquitous Computing and Virtual Reality that Influence Nursing Education and Practice

- All nurses will need to have some degree of computer literacy: the ability not only to understand computers but also to use them effectively and apply the knowledge gained.
- Ubiquitous computing (UC) extends the "PC Era," which essentially means one person per (personal) computer. In the UC phase, computers move from the realm of personal application to one of computers being fundamental, everyday items. Microprocessors are already in many objects throughout the house, including microwaves, TV remotes, and appliances. With UC, the application of the computer becomes commonplace, but the computerization itself fades into the background.
- Virtual reality (VR) is the active application of a computer-generated world in which "what if" scenarios can be simulated. Medicine has developed many surgical techniques using VR, with medical and nursing education offering training in using some of these applications.
- VR can assist students and patients alike in understanding clinical procedures. For example, if a patient is about to undergo a procedure, he can "watch" it via computer, which offers the nurse an educational opportunity with the patient not only to ensure that the procedure is understood but also to review the care that will be needed before and after the procedure.
- The Internet continues to change the way that professionals as well as patients obtain information. Today, patients are much more informed because of the wealth of knowledge available on the Internet. It is the health care provider's responsibility, however, to ensure that the information they receive is accurate and applicable to their particular situation.

Applying Criteria to Evaluating Internet Sites

- The purpose-focus-approach assessment (Nicoll, 2003) is one method to apply when evaluating Internet sites. During the first step (purpose), you need to identify why you are conducting the search. The purpose of your search then leads you to a focus of basic or technical, professional or patient-oriented.
- Quick and dirty searching can use a general search engine (e.g., Google or Dogpile). You will generally receive many "hits" and can then begin to narrow your focus.
- Brute-force searching is when you simply type in what you believe to be the address, using the probable domain name.
- Links and bookmarks can be used effectively to narrow your results once you have completed a quick and dirty or a brute force search.
- Always keep a listing of well-known, well-researched sites that can be used as starting points.
- Literature resources include MEDLINE, National Guideline Clearinghouse, and others.
- Use the mnemonic PLEASED to evaluate websites. P: Purpose of the site is clear? L: Links are active and working? E: Editorial issues of clarity of writing and site content are addressed? A: Author is clearly identified, with appropriate credentials? S: Site is easy to navigate and attractive? E: Ethical disclosure of the author and site developer is made? D: Date the site was last updated is provided?

CASE SCENARIOS

Guided Case Scenario 4-1

You are the nursing supervisor for a 3-11 shift. While making rounds one evening, you come upon a small grouping of critical care nurses around the centralized computer, and you overhear some of their conversation. They are discussing a colleague who was newly diagnosed with AIDS and a sexually transmitted disease. You find out that their colleague is a patient on one of the medical-surgical units and that the nurses found this out as they were scanning the patient listings in the hospital. In fact, this particular group of nurses regularly scans the inpatient listing to see if they know anyone.

Case Considerations

1. What is your first response, as a supervisor, to this situation?
2. What are the parameters for seeing confidential information on a computer system at work?
3. What is the next step for you, as a supervisor, to take?

Case Analysis

1. What is your first response, as a supervisor, to this situation?

Breach of confidentiality is a serious offense, regardless of the medium involved or the person who is breaking this trust. Every patient has a right to confidentially and to know that his or her medical and health care information is secure. Security measures need to be in place to assure that the integrity of the data as well as compliance with federal and state laws and regulations are maintained. Access should be granted only to those who are authorized and have a justifiable reason for viewing the data.

Seeing staff members huddled around a computer and scanning for people they may know who have been admitted to the hospital is a serious breach of privacy and confidentiality for the patients involved. The supervisor should take immediate action with the staff nurses and follow protocol in informing their immediate supervisor.

2. What are the parameters for seeing confidential information on a computer system at work?

Confidential information involves the act of limiting who sees private information. All health care providers have the moral and legal responsibility to maintain confidentiality of information that is considered private. Even if you may not think a particular piece of information would be considered something that needs to be kept private, a patient should expect that all information, regardless of the content, is private.

3. What is the next step for you, as a supervisor, to take?

Most institutions have in-depth policies for maintaining confidentiality and security of health information as well as policies for working with electronic data and informatics. At the point of discovery, you should, at the least, verbally reprimand the staff, document the event, and follow up as appropriate. The Risk Manager and, perhaps, the Chief Information Officer of the facility also need to be brought into the discussion of this serious breach of patient confidentially.

Case Scenario 4-2

You are the lead nurse on a busy oncology unit, and you have been a nurse for more than 30 years. The Medical Director seeks you out one day and says that he would like to begin a new form of art therapy to lift the patients' spirits. He remembers reading about the therapy "in some magazine somewhere," but he is not sure what the magazine was or what month the article was published. All he remembers is that the article was in a magazine or journal, that it was specifically about art therapy in hospitals, and that he thinks it may have mentioned something about oncology patients. He asks you to find the article, because he just met someone influential who is willing to donate the funds to begin the project. Unfortunately, you are not computer savvy; in fact, all you really know how to do on a computer is retrieve the laboratory values and do order entry. You are not quite sure where to begin.

Case Considerations

1. You can begin your search for the art therapy article in several ways, but the easiest is to use the computer. Where do you start?
2. List several strategies for searching the Internet.
3. What is the purpose-focus-approach assessment, and how can you apply it to your search?
4. Other methods for searching the Internet include quick and dirty as well as brute force searching. What are these methods, and how are they different?
5. Knowing that you are looking for information specific to oncology patients, what are some possible resources to search on this topic?
6. After you have exhausted all the nonprofessional sources, you turn to the literature resources for the professional reader. Identify some of these sources, and explain how you would use them in your search.
7. How would you begin to evaluate whether the journal article's findings are valid and applicable?

Case Analysis

Although it may seem like it, not everyone has the same comfort level with the computer or with accessing information on it. If you were this lead nurse's manager, how could you alleviate her anxiety so that she could complete the request by the physician? Are there any classes at the hospital in which you can enroll her? Are there any computer educators on staff who may be able to assist her?

■ *KEY POINTS*

1. The Internet is used for a variety of reasons, including information gathering and retrieval. Not all the information found on the Internet, however, is accurate or current, and you need a critical eye to evaluate it.
2. A website can be evaluated in several ways, with the PLEASED mnemonic being a helpful choice.
3. PubMed is a vast search engine developed by the National Library of Medicine. With PubMed, one can search many journals in the MEDLARS system, offering professional and laypeople alike access to medical, nursing, and other health care information.
4. Colleges and universities that offer a health major will have extensive professional literature, both in hard-copy journal as well as electronic format.

References

American Nurses Association. (1994). *Scope of practice for nursing informatics.* Washington, D.C.: American Nurses Publishing.

Nicoll, S. (2003). Nursing and health care informatics. In P. Kelly-Heidenthal (Ed.), *Nursing leadership and management* (pp. 75–96), Clifton Park, NY: Delmar Learning.

Suggested Readings

Ball, M., Hannah, K. J., Newbold, S., & Douglas, J. (2000). *Nursing informatics: Where caring and technology meet* (3rd ed.). New York: Springer-Verlag.

Bozak, M. G. (2003). Using Lewin's force field analysis in implementing a nursing information system. *Computers, Informatics, Nursing, 21* (2), 80–87.

Cader, R., Campbell, S., & Watson, D. (2003). Criteria used by nurses to evaluate practice-related information on the World Wide Web. *Computers, Informatics, Nursing, 21* (2), 97–102.

Chastain, A. R. (2003). Nursing informatics: Past, present and future. *Tennessee Nurse, 66* (1), 8–10.

Fairey, M. (2003). Miss Nightingale was right. *British Journal of Healthcare Computing & Information Management, 20* (1), 3.

Hebda, T., Czar, P., & Mascara, C. (1998). *Handbook of informatics for nurses and health care professionals.* Menlo Park, CA: Addison-Wesley.

Kinn, S., & Doucherty, C. (2003). Issues for research in nursing informatics. *British Journal of Healthcare Computing & Information Management, 20* (1), 23–25.

Kongstvedt, P. (2002). *Managed care: What it is and how it works.* Gaithersburg, MD: Aspen Publishers.

Maddock, E. (2002). The benefits of implementing an electronic patient record system. *Nursing Times, 98* (49), 34–36.

McDaniel, A. M. (2003). Using technology to advance the knowledge work of clinical nurse specialists: Part I, organizing data. *Clinical Nurse Specialist, 17* (2), 78–80.

Newbold, S. (1996). The informatics nurse and the certification process. *Computers in Nursing, 14* (2), 84–85, 88.

Nicoll, L. H. (2000). *Nurses' guide to the Internet* (3rd ed.). Philadelphia: Lippincott Williams & Wilkins.

Olsen, L. (2003). Privacy and confidentiality in an electronic age. *Chart, 100* (1), 9.

Romano, C. A., Mills, M. E., & Heller, B. R. (1996). *Information management in nursing and health care.* Springhouse, PA: Springhouse.

Rossel, C. L. (2003). HIPPA: An informatics system perspective. *Chart, 100* (1), 11.

Saba, V. K. (2002). Home health care classification system (HHCS): An overview. *Online Journal of Issues in Nursing, 7* (3), 22.

Young, K. M. (2000). *Informatics for healthcare professionals.* Philadelphia: F. A. Davis.

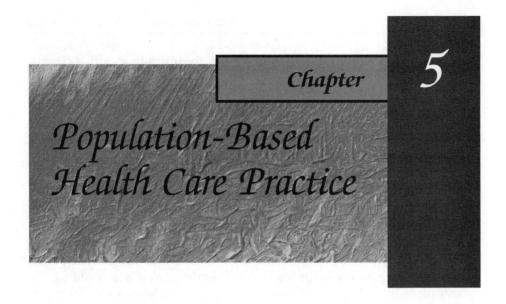

Chapter 5

Population-Based Health Care Practice

Essential Concepts in Population-Based Health Care Practice

The notion of population-based health care is not new; nurses have been working in the community since nursing began as a profession. The focus of population-based health care is the advocacy of those people who are at greatest risk for a poor health status based on access to quality care, whether because of cost, availability, or other barriers, such as language, lack of transportation, or lack of education and knowledge.

A predominant focus of population-based health care is health promotion and disease prevention. Many vulnerable populations have chronic health problems. They may seek medical care only when they absolutely have to, however, and by that time, the chronic condition has not only exacerbated, it may be confounded by a new, acute condition. Population-based nursing care is holistic in nature, with nurses attempting to understand the client from a variety of perspectives, including socioeconomic, cultural, racial, religious, gender, abilities, and sexual affiliation. The application of the nursing process greatly assists the nurse in providing holistic care on the community, health systems, and population levels.

Social Initiatives to Provide Population-Based Care

- Population-based care is the "development, provision and evaluation of the multidisciplinary health care services to population groups experiencing increased health risks or disparities" (Schoon, 2003, p. 98). Population-based care works closely and collaboratively with community and health care team members to maintain or improve the health of all the diverse members who make up a community.
- Communities often have vulnerable population groups who are disadvantaged in terms of health care access or issues of cost or quality.
- These discrepancies in care may result in decreased health status and place the members of these communities at higher risk for developing a complicated health status, in which morbidity and mortality are increased.
- One model used extensively to determine the health of a particular community is the Healthy People in Healthy Communities 2010 model (Figure 5-1), which delineates four elements needed to achieve health improvement: goals, objectives, determinants of health, and health status.
- Social mandates to improve health care status are found at the community, state, regional, national, and global levels. For example, infant mortality rates in the United States are among the highest for developed countries, with every state attempting to decrease these rates through a variety of programs and initiatives (Table 5-1).

Practice of Population-Based Nursing

- The practice of population-based nursing has existed since the founding of the nursing profession, beginning with Florence Nightingale.
- Population-based health care focuses on specific groups of people (hence the "population") and applies health promotion and disease prevention methodologies. A prevailing goal of population-based nursing care is to improve the overall health status of the identified community.
- Population-based care is holistic in nature, considering not only the physiologic concerns of the patient but also ethnic, cultural, psychological, spiritual, economic, and gender differences.
- A vulnerable population is one that is often underserved by medical care services. An example would be the migrant farm workers from

A Systematic Approach to Health Improvement

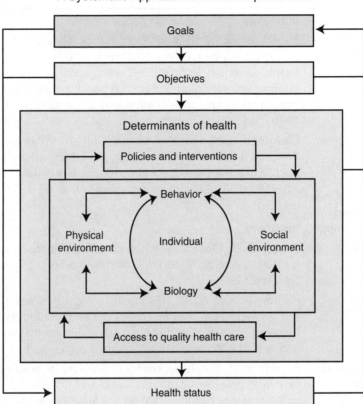

Figure 5-1   Healthy People 2001. Retrieved January 20, 2002, from
               http://www.health.gov

Mexico, who have little access to area health care services in the
United States because of issues of transportation, language, culture,
money, and knowledge. Many traditional acute care facilities do not
have options to treat patients on an ongoing preventative basis,
which is one reason why many vulnerable peoples have high
emergency department utilization rates.
• A community assessment is generally the starting point for
  population-based nursing care, with a consideration for
  multidisciplinary input and services.

Population-Based Planning and Evaluation Process

• The components of the population-based planning and evaluation
  process are similar to those of the nursing process components,

Table 5-1 Population-Based Health Care Initiatives

Global Group	Initiatives
World Health Organization	Health for All by the Year 2000. Principles delineated in the Health for All by the Year 2000 plan include (1) the right to health, (2) equity in health, (3) community participation, (4) intersectoral collaboration, (5) health promotion, (6) primary health care, and (7) international cooperation (Bastian, 1989, p. 15).
United Nations	Cairo Action Plan for Women's Health. This plan illustrates the clear link between education, poverty, gender equality, culture, national politics and economies, population growth, and the health status of women (Nelson, et al., 1996).

National and Regional Group	Initiatives
Great Britain	Saving Lives: Our Healthier Nation. This initiative focused on the prevention of 300,000 deaths in a 10-year period (Mitchell, 1999).
United States	Healthy People 2010. This initiative highlights health indicators related to the leading causes of death, including health behaviors, physical and social and environmental factors, and health systems factors. (Healthy People, n. d.).
American Public Association (APHA)	Recommends the development of a universal health care system to provide for the uninsured and disenfranchised of the country. Commentary on the State of the Public's Health (American Public Health Association, 2001).

State	Initiatives
Arizona	Tobacco Education and Prevention Program (TEPP) (Centers for Disease Control, 2001).
Arkansas	Community-oriented primary care (COPC) model utilizing family nurse practitioners (Hartwig & Landis, 1999).
New Hampshire	The New Hampshire Coalition against Domestic and Sexual Violence (Hastings, 2001).
New Mexico	"Roll up Your Sleeves" campaign to combat the high incidence of hepatitis B in the state's population (Harris, Kerr, & Steffen, 1997).
Tennessee	Tenncare, a program to extend health care benefits to the uninsured and to slow down the rapid growth of Medicaid spending (Lyons & Scheb, 1998).

which are assessment, nursing diagnosis, planning, implementation, and evaluation.

- Community level assessments for population-based planning and evaluation include the physical and social environment and policies and interventions.
- Health system level assessments for population-based planning and evaluation include access to quality health care.
- Population level assessments for population-based planning and evaluation include biological, behavioral, and data analysis of the at-risk population as well as identification of the health risks of the population.

CASE SCENARIOS

Guided Case Scenario 5-1

You volunteer at a free neighborhood health clinic one night a week. The vast majority of your patients come from the migrant farms in the area. Most are immigrants from Mexico and do not speak English. The clinic sees adults primarily, but many times, parents will also bring their sick children to be seen by the doctor or nurse. No pediatric free clinic is available.

The line for the clinic begins well before its doors open. Many are turned away when the clinic is open, simply because there are more who need to be seen than there are hours in which to see them. The clinic is small, with only a few examination rooms, one waiting room, and one medication room. Medications are donated by local physicians or pharmacies. Patients pay on a sliding scale.

The health problems of the patients vary, with a wide range of chronic and acute diseases. The vast majority of patients suffer from complications of diabetes, hypertension, alcoholism, and obesity. Unfortunately, some have no other access to health care, because they are in this country illegally and, therefore, are not eligible for American health care benefits. Money is an issue with all who come to the clinic, as is transportation, sufficient housing, access to educational facilities, language, and adequate nutrition.

Case Considerations

1. Given the four primary diseases that are seen in the clinic, what are the contributing social and environmental factors?

2. Identify at least four modifiable risk factors that you, as a nurse, can address.
3. What are the three levels of population-based assessment, and how can they be applied to this population of predominately migrant workers?
4. What are some data sources for assisting you in the population-based assessment?
5. If you were given the opportunity to write a grant proposal for improving the health care of the clinic population, on what area would you focus and why?
6. What type of nursing leadership opportunities could you seek out in this setting?

Case Analysis

1. Given the four primary diseases that are seen in the clinic, what are the contributing social and environmental factors?

   Diabetes, hypertension, alcoholism, and obesity are the four most common diseases that are seen in the clinic. All four can be hereditary, but they can also be brought on by influencing environmental and social factors. Some of these influencing factors could be poor nutrition: If the foods consumed are high in calories, fat, and salt and have low nutritional value, obesity and hypertension could result. In turn, diabetes can result from obesity. Alcoholism may be exacerbated by boredom, lack of self-esteem, and other social factors. Stress may contribute to the development of alcoholism and hypertension.

2. Identify at least four modifiable risk factors that you, as a nurse, can address.

   Nonmodifiable risk factors are age, gender, ethnicity, and race. Modifiable risk factors are those variables that affect and can cause changes in an individual's health status. In this population, modifiable risk factors could be the social and physical environment, educational issues, hereditary issues, stress and other psychosocial concerns, and lack of adequate medical care.

3. What are the three levels of population-based assessment, and how can they be applied to this population of predominately migrant workers?

   Population-based assessment begins at the community level, where the physical environment, the social environment, and policies and interventions are the key areas. Housing, the community, transportation, and the school system are some of the identified areas in the physical environment, along with the basic environmental qualities. The social environment not only looks at the culture, values, and societal norms of the community but also at its safety and employment opportunities. Although this community is in the United States and, therefore, is governed by American policies and interventions, each community handles its own problems, with its individual city and social policies. Other systems have certain policies and procedures that the community accepts, such as health care access, transportation access, and even basic communications.

The health systems level is primarily concerned with access to quality health care at the primary, secondary and tertiary levels. It can be assumed from the case scenario that such access in this community is lacking, especially if many who need basic, primary care are turned away each time the clinic doors open. How far out of town is the hospital located? How do the workers enter the health care system if they do not have insurance? What do their children do for basic medical care?

The last level is the population level, in which one reviews the data from a more generalized viewpoint rather than from an individual town or city. Data such as demographics, along with biological patterns of health and illness, are kept. Behavioral issues, such as educational levels, socioeconomic status, cultural patterns, and health patterns, are reviewed as part of the assessment phase. Finally, the data analysis prioritizes the health needs of the community by reviewing the risk factors found in the community.

4. What are some data sources for assisting you in the population-based assessment?

Primary data can be collected in a variety of ways and using a variety of methods. The easiest way to collect data is simply to observe the community at work, at rest, and at play. Other methods include interviewing key informants, who often are civic leaders, religious leaders, and governmental officials, as well as a cross-section of the population. Secondary data are those that you do not necessarily collect yourself; they include a variety of sources, such as vital statistics, planning documents, reports, a review of the literature, and local and community news sources.

5. If you were given the opportunity to write a grant proposal for improving the health care of the clinic population, on what area would you focus and why?

   This clinic population could benefit from just about any type of intervention. You would want to perform an in-depth population-based assessment and, depending on your findings, focus your grant application on that particular data. Are there issues in the physical or social environment? Is there an issue with access to quality health care? Are there modifiable health risk factors?

   You may want to focus on certain barriers, such as language, cultural differences, lack of health information, education, access to care, or many others. Because the town does not have a pediatric clinic, would there be a need? Is there a need for focused interventions on one of the four primary diseases seen in the clinic?

6. What type of nursing leadership opportunities could you seek out in this setting?

   There are so many leadership opportunities in this clinic environment that all you need to do is simply choose an area of interest. If you speak Spanish, you could be a lead interpreter, could offer medical classes in Spanish for the health care providers and staff, or could offer English classes for the patients. If grantsmanship is one of your strengths, you could aggressively seek those opportunities to complement the limited budget and finances. If you have strong mentoring skills, you could work with the new volunteers, preparing them in the ways of the clinic and working with them until they are comfortable in their new environment. Depending on the medical or nursing needs, you could offer specific classes for the clients. Numerous leadership opportunities exist in this type of volunteer environment; all you need to do is to look and decide where to focus your energies.

Case Scenario 5-2

You just recently took a new position in the health department as a public health nurse. You begin your rounds with Mr. Perrier, who was discharged from the hospital several days ago with status post right foot amputation because of complications from diabetes. On entering his home, you notice that all the blinds are drawn; that the air is musty, with a fetid odor coming from a corner of the room; and that an elderly man is sitting at the kitchen table.

Mr. Perrier does not have any relatives to assist him with dressing changes, and his current dressing looks as if it has not been changed since his discharge from the hospital. Mr. Perrier does not speak much English and is native to Haiti. He looks like he is in discomfort, does not make much eye contact with you, and makes no real attempt to communicate.

Case Considerations

1. What are some of the primary issues, other than his wound care, surrounding Mr. Perrier?
2. Identify several of his health risk factors.
3. What are his instrumental activities of daily living?
4. How would you determine his functional health status and ability to perform his activities of daily living?
5. What are the nursing and medical priorities for Mr. Perrier? How should one proceed with this first visit? What should the plans be for subsequent visits?
6. Identify social and other issues, other than the obvious health-related ones, that may complicate Mr. Perrier's healing process.

Case Analysis

Like many patients who are considered to be part of a vulnerable community, Mr. Perrier is dealing with numerous issues in addition to the catastrophic event of his foot amputation. When providing population-based health care, a nurse can always apply the nursing process as a basis for nursing care delivery. Many times, we want to address only the health-related issue. In this case, to provide holistic care the entire person needs to be considered as being of equal importance to the specific health-related issue, as do his social, religious and cultural considerations.

■ KEY POINTS

1. A person's environment is critical to achieving health. Identify some of the barriers in Mr. Perrier's environment. What can be done to change these barriers? How can one assist Mr. Perrier in understanding that these barriers are truly health concerns?

In looking at Mr. Perrier's health risk factors, how important is it that he speaks English?

2. How does one determine his instrumental activities of daily living? His functional health status? His ability to perform his activities of daily living?

3. What is the first priority for Mr. Perrier? How often does a home health nurse need to visit him? Discuss the next three priorities of Mr. Perrier's care. How many of these priorities are health-related?

4. Are there any community resources that one may be able to engage in Mr. Perrier's care? What should the expectations be of these community resources? Are there any other resources that may be able to assist Mr. Perrier in achieving optimal health?

References

American Public Health Association. (2001). *The fourteen points for the campaign for universal health care—the nation's health.* http://www.apha.org

Bastian, H. (1989). A guide to WHO and "WHO speak." *Consumer Health Forum,* 9, 15.

Centers for Disease Control. (2001). Tobacco use among adults—Arizona, 1996 and 1999. *Morbidity and Mortality Weekly Report, 50* (20), 402–406. Retrieved March 27, 2002, from http://www.cdc.gov

Harris, P. A., Kerr, J. & Steffen, D. (1997). A state-based immunization campaign: the New Mexico experience. *Journal of School Health, 67* (7), 272–276.

Hartwig, M. S. & Landis, B. J. (1999). The Arkansas AHEC model of community-oriented primary care. *Holistic Nurse Practitioner,* 13(4), 28–37.

Hastings, D. P. (2001). The New Hampshire health initiative on domestic violence. *Nursing Forum,* 36(1), 31–35.

Lyons, W. & Scheb, J. M. II. (1998). Managed care and Medicaid reform in Tennessee: The impact of Tenncare on access and health-seeking behavior. *Journal of Health Care for the Poor and Underserved,* 10(3), 328–337.

Mitchell, P. (1999). UK government aims to prevent 300,000 deaths over ten years. *Lancet,* 354, 139.

Nelson, M., Proctor, S., Regev, H., Barnes, D., Sawyer, L., Messias, D., Yoder, L., & Meleis, A. I. (1996). International population and development: The United Nations' Cairo action plan for women's health. *Image: Journal of Nursing Scholarship,* 28(1), 75–80.

Schoon, P. M. (2003). Population-based health care practice. In P. Kelly-Heidenthal (Ed.), *Nursing leadership and management* (pp. 97–118), Clifton Park, NY: Delmar Learning.

U.S. Department of Health and Human Services. (2000). *Healthy people 2010: Understanding and improving health* (2nd ed.). Washington, DC: U.S. Government Printing Office.

Suggested Readings

Baldwin, J. H., Conger, C. O., Abegglen, J. C., & Hill, E. M. (1998). Population-focused and community-based nursing—Moving toward clarification of concepts. *Public Health Nursing, 15* (1), 12–18.

Beauchesne, M. F. (2001). When urban U.S. means urban underserved. *Reflections on Nursing Leadership, 27* (2), 24–27.

Green, P. M., & Slade, D. S. (2000). Environmental nursing diagnoses for aggregates and Community. *Nursing Diagnosis, 12* (1), 5–13.

Keller, L. O., Strohschein, S., Lia-Hoagberg, B., & Schafer, M. (1998). Population-based public health nursing interventions: A model from practice. *Public Health Nursing, 15* (3), 207–215.

Kongstvedt, P. (2001). *Essentials in managed care* (4th ed.). Gaithersburg, MD: Aspen Publishers.

Kurland, J. (2000). Public health in the new millennium. II: Social exclusion. *Public Health Reports, 115* (4), 298.

Meisenheimer, C. G. (1997). *Improving quality.* Gaithersburg, MD: Aspen Publishers.

O'Neil, E. H., & the Pew Health Professions Commission. (1998). *Recreating health professional practice for a new century.* San Francisco: Pew Health Professions Commission.

Shui, L., & Singh, D. A. (1998). *Delivering health care in America.* Gaithersburg, MD: Aspen Publishers.

Stanhope, M., & Lancaster, J. (1996). *Community health nursing: Process and practice for promoting health.* St. Louis, MO: Mosby–Year Book.

U.S. Department of Health and Human Services. (2001). *Healthy people 2010: Goals.* Retrieved June 16, 2003, from http://www.health.gov

Wolper, L. (1999). *Health care administration planning, implementing and managing organized delivery systems* (3rd ed.). Gaithersburg, MD: Aspen Publishers.

Chapter 6

Personal and Interdisciplinary Communication

Essential Concepts in Personal and Interdisciplinary Communication

Effective communication is probably the most valuable tool that any manager can possess, and it is the core of any management activity. Organizational communication occurs at all levels of management and includes both written and verbal expertise. There are as many techniques for establishing and maintaining valuable communication skills as there are strategies for assisting managers and staff alike in overcoming the multiple barriers that one encounters daily in both the workplace and home.

Nurses engage in communications that are vertical, horizontal, lateral, and diagonal—sometimes during the same conversation. Differing communication styles are learned when dealing with patients and their families and with physicians and other professionals, as well as in different situations and settings. Issues such as gender, the organizational hierarchy, and the informal grapevine may affect the adequacy of both sending and receiving the message accurately. Both formal and informal networks of interaction need to be recognized as contributing to complex communication patterns. It is critical that managers and staff at all levels understand this potential for misunderstandings within the organization.

Trends in Society that Affect Communication

- Several trends in the United States affect communication patterns. These include the aging population, increasing diversity, differing values and belief sets, and increasing reliance on computers and other technology.

Elements of the Communication Process

- An effective communication process has four key elements: the sender, the actual message, the receiver of the message, and the feedback regarding what the receiver truly heard.

Modes of Communication

- Verbal communications use the spoken word to send and receive messages and are critically dependent on the four elements of the communication process.
- Nonverbal communications take into account all means of communications, including facial and body gesturing.
- Electronic communications include the technologies to get the spoken word across and include computers, voice mail, and e-mail.

Increasing Effective Communication Skills

- To enhance communication skills nurses need, in addition to the four elements of the communication process, to be aware of several skills that will increase mutual understanding.
- Attending is potentially the most important skill to acquire, and it consists of practicing active listening.
- Responding is a key element of feedback. It consists of both verbal and nonverbal acknowledgement of a received communication.
- Clarifying is used when there is a need to ensure clarity in the message both being sent and received.
- Confronting is when the messenger or receiver asks for clarification to jointly resolve an issue or concern.
- Using open-ended questions, rather than asking for a yes or no response, often gives the most opportunity for receivers of a message to express themselves.

Barriers to Effective Communication

- Men and women often have different communication styles and patterns, so gender often gets in the way of effective and mutual understanding.
- Culture, in the expressed differences of language, values, beliefs, dress, and nonverbal expectations, may lead to unintentional misunderstandings.
- Anger is often a barrier to effective communication.
- Often, what one says is not what one means; in other words, the verbal message is not the same as the nonverbal message. These are considered to be incongruent responses.
- Different people have different ways of dealing with conflict. Avoidance occurs when the person retreats from the situation. Accommodation occurs when the needs of others take priority over your own. Competition occurs when one person wins and the other loses, whereas compromise results when both sides give up something important. The best strategy to encourage effective communication patterns is to establish a collaborative style, in which both sides are satisfied with the offered solution.

CASE SCENARIOS

Guided Case Scenario 6-1

You are the manager of a telemetry unit at a hospital that has seasonal variations because of tourists visiting during the winter months. As a result of the variability in patient census, the hospital cannot keep all the units open year-round and depends on the flexibility of staff and managers alike to be creative when the census is high and bed availability is minimal. During the past winter season, patients were often kept in the Emergency Department for a day or two until a bed opened up on the medical-surgical floors, resulting in many upset patients, staff, and physicians.

Your Chief Nursing Officer (CNO) recently received approval from the Chief Executive Officer (CEO) to open an ancillary unit out of a space that was once occupied by the Physical Therapy Department but is now empty. She asks you to supervise the opening of the unit as well as the staffing. She is willing to approve several travelers for this unit, but you know that your staff may also be interested in the temporary unit. This is the first unit of its type for the hospital, and realizing that that the potential for misunder-standing its purpose, the patient population, and who staffs the unit is high, you begin your planning.

Case Considerations

1. Who are the key individuals that should be in the communication loop, and why are they chosen?
2. What are the different methods of communicating to the above-mentioned individuals? How would one chose the most effective method for each group, and why?
3. A timeline needs to be established for opening the unit. How would one establish and communicate this timeline to others? Who should be involved with its development?
4. How would the nurse manager handle the situation if some staff were openly antagonist about the new unit, because it may mean that they are responsible for providing staffing coverage?

Case Analysis

1. Who are the key individuals that should be in the communication loop, and why are they chosen?

A hospital system contains complex communication loops, both formal and informal. Once the CNO and the CEO have decided to establish this ancillary unit and you have been designated as the responsible manager, there needs to be a plan for communicating the news along with the other, more fundamental issues of staffing, resource procurement, and admission, discharge, and transfer criteria for the patients.

The first step is to communicate, both verbally and in writing, to all the stakeholders of the unit. Stakeholders include the telemetry staff, potential per-diem staff, physicians, the staffing office, nursing supervisors, and other patient care areas within the hospital. You can present the new unit information at your staff meetings, ensuring that minutes are kept and available for those staff members who are not able to attend. A memo could be distributed to all key managers and physicians in the facility, and all the patient care units could receive a copy. The telemetry's medical director would need to have this knowledge as well and, in turn, would be able to take that information to the telemetry medical staff via their monthly meetings.

2. What are the different methods of communicating to the above-mentioned individuals? How would one chose the most effective method for each group, and why?

The most common method would be one-to-one conversations. This is also, however, the most tedious method. In addition, it has the most potential for misunderstanding, because one would be repeating the same message frequently. Having the conversation in a group setting is helpful, because numerous people hear the same message at the same time, which decreases the potential for misinterpretation.

A memo is efficient and, when well written, can clear up most misperceptions. The memo can be sent via e-mail to many people at one time, saving paper and expense. If someone does not have e-mail capacity—and many staff nurses do not—the manager can print a hard copy of a memo and post it. Also helpful is to have those who have read the memo initial it.

For the physician group, several methods may have to be used to have the majority of them receive the message. Many physicians have e-mail capacity, but an office manager, not the physician, may be the actual person taking off a message. Discussion of the unit change at a staff meeting, followed by a memo to their mailbox at the hospital and, perhaps, an e-mail message, would ensure that most physicians would receive this message.

3. A timeline needs to be established for opening the unit. How would one establish and communicate this timeline to others? Who should be involved with its development?

The staff are probably the most essential personnel to work with in establishing the new unit. To encourage them to "buy in" to the proposal, they should be included as early as the planning phase of the unit. Begin by ensuring that all staff know of this new unit, whether personally, through a staff meeting, or by memo. Once the initial information has been disseminated, it would be helpful for any questions to be answered, either in a staff meeting, on an information sheet (with a title similar to "Questions and Answers"), or even on a poster board that outlines the progress.

4. How would the nurse manager handle the situation if some staff were openly antagonist about the new unit, because it may mean that they are responsible for providing staffing coverage?

Hopefully, all staff have been in the information loop from the beginning (once the decision has been made to open the ancillary unit). Not all staff will be pleased with the new unit, however, because it means floating to the new unit and, sometimes, going shorter-staffed on the telemetry unit to accommodate the new unit. If you hear of staff members who are negative, it is best to confront them immediately. Perhaps they have incorrect information, and all they need is someone to provide the facts. Maybe they are listening to the informal grapevine, which usually contains some truth to the message but may be inaccurate or misleading overall. Again, it is imperative to address these issues early on with staff, before the incorrect information gets to more people outside the unit. One does not want the new unit to fail even before it has a chance to succeed, especially because of rumors, bad will, or inaccurate information. Finally, if certain staff continue to have negative attitudes about the new unit, perhaps it may be time to begin a different tact, such as mentoring and counseling.

Case Scenario 6-2

You are the coordinator of a clinic in a health department. Jason is the lead registered nurse (RN) on the day shift and has been for 3 years. He carries one of the heaviest caseloads of any of your nurses and has always received high evaluations from clients. Because this is a small clinic, generally only three RNs are assigned to any one shift. It is now August, and it will soon be time for the student nurses to return to the clinic. They have been using your agency as a clinical practice site for the last year. Six students are assigned at a time to work in the agency, and you generally assign two students per nurse.

Several students have reported bad experiences working with Jason. They say that he openly ignores them in front of clients, and they believe that he destroys any rapport or credibility they might otherwise have with the clients. He rolls his eyes when a student offers suggestions, or he crosses his hands across his chest, giving them the impression that he is not interested in their input. They say he belittles the charting they do, and when their instructor is not present, he tells them to "go back to the simulation lab where you belong." The nursing instructor does not want to "get involved" and has asked you to intervene with Jason.

Case Considerations

1. What nonverbal behaviors is Jason exhibiting and communicating to the students? To the patients?
2. As the coordinator of the clinic, what methods could you employ to assist Jason with improving his communication?
3. Will you say anything to the nursing students? How will you respond to the nursing instructor?
4. What are some alternative actions to ensure that the students have a good experience? Explain some actions to take with Jason.
5. What might be some educational opportunities for Jason?

Case Analysis

In reviewing this case, you realize that both verbal and nonverbal issues surround Jason, the staff, the nursing students, and the instructor. It is imperative that you, as a manager, get all sides of the story before assuming that one party is causing all the difficulty.

■ KEY POINTS

1. Nonverbal communications sometimes contain stronger messages than verbal communications. Think of some of the issues that can arise from Jason's nonverbal behavior.
2. There may be unintentional messages that are transmitted by the students and instructor during their interactions with the clinic nurses and with Jason. How could the students be contributing to the situation?
3. Sometimes communication misunderstandings simply need to be discussed by the parties involved in an open and safe environment. Would a session such as this be appropriate to solve this issue? What might the potential problems be if this session is not handled correctly?
4. How could the clinic coordinator help Jason before the students arrive in the clinic? Sometimes, people are not aware of how they communicate, especially to subordinates, and they may need guidance and mentoring.

Case Scenario 6-3

As the nurse manager, you are completing your rounds one morning when you stop by and introduce yourself to Mrs. Frenne, an elderly and frail woman with congestive heart failure. She has nothing but praise for the staff, the medical care, and the hospital—except for one nursing assistant, Annie, who has been assigned to her for the last three days in a row. A new employee, Annie just received her certified nursing assistance certificate after moving to the United States from Jamaica several months ago. She appears to be competent. Her mannerisms are sometimes abrupt, however, and she avoids direct eye contact.

When you ask Mrs. Frenne what the issue is, she states that the nursing assistant speaks to her harshly, in a stern voice. Just this morning, the nursing assistant told Mrs. Frenne in an abrupt tone that she had to get out of bed and walk, because "it was good for her." Not wanting to antagonize the nursing assistant, Mrs. Frenne walked the length of the corridor and is now quite short of breath. This is the second patient that has complained about Annie's tone of voice and her stern way of communicating.

Case Considerations

1. As the manager, what would be your first reaction to this scenario? Is Mrs. Frenne believable? Why, or why not?
2. As the manager, what can you do to make Mrs. Frenne feel better about her recovery on this unit?
3. Why should a manager care about a patient's satisfaction with the staff?
4. Discuss some possible ways to remedy this situation between Mrs. Frenne and the nursing assistant.
5. How could the nursing assistant better communicate with Mrs. Frenne in particular and with other patients in general? Identify the nonverbal messages that are communicated by the nursing assistant.

Case Analysis

One of the most important functions of a nurse manager is making rounds on the patients in the unit. Rounds give the manager an opportunity to meet the patients, to assess their progress, and to gain a general understanding about their level of satisfaction with the nursing care and their hospitalization. Rounds also give the manager a chance to turn a negative experience into a positive one before the patient is discharged. It appears that an opportunity may exist in this scenario to "turn around" a damaging situation before Mrs. Frenne is discharged by getting the nursing assistant to apologize.

■ KEY POINTS

1. Having a manager speak with a patient can clear up a misunderstanding between the patient and a staff member. Often, patients and their families simply want to be reassured that their issues are "heard" and that someone takes an interest in their well-being.
2. Assuming that this was not an isolated incident of poor communication by Annie, what are some issues to keep in mind as you plan your meeting with her to discuss Mrs. Frenne's concerns? There are many factors to consider with Annie, including a new position, a new career, and possibly, cultural differences in communication styles.
3. One significant role of a manager is staff development and coaching of both new and experienced employees. What is the appropriate plan for Annie?

Suggested Readings

Armstrong, L., & McKenchnie, K. (2003). Intergenerational communication. *International Journal of Language & Communication Disorders, 38* (1), 13–29.

Bayne, C. G. (1997). Speak to me! An overview of patient communication. *Nursing Management, 28* (4), 48–52.

Bellack, J. P., & O'Neil, E. H. (2000). Recreating nursing practice for a new century. *Nursing and Health Care Perspectives, 21* (1), 15–21.

Cioffi, R. N. J. (2003). Communicating with culturally and linguistically diverse patients in an acute care setting: Nurses' experiences. *International Journal of Nursing Studies, 40* (3), 299–306.

DiBartola, L. (2001). Listening to your patients and responding with care. *Joint Commission Journal on Quality Improvement, 27* (6), 315–323.

Healthcare Education Associates. (1988). *Professional writing skills for health care managers: A practical guide.* St. Louis, MO: C. V. Mosby.

Henderson, E. (2003). Communication and managerial effectiveness. *Nursing Management (London), 9* (9): 30–34

Luckman, J. (1999). *Transcultural communication in nursing.* New York: Delmar Publications.

Marquis, B. L., & Huston, C. J. (2000). *Leadership roles and management functions* (3rd ed.). Philadelphia: J. B. Lippincott.

Parsons, L. C. (2002). Transcultural communication: The cornerstone to transcultural care. *SCI Nursing, 19* (4), 160, 162–163.

Rocchiccioli, J. T., & Tilbury, M. S. (1998). *Clinical leadership in nursing.* Philadelphia: W. B. Saunders.

Sellers, S. (1991). *Language and sexual differences.* London: Macmillan.

Shaffer, B., Tallarica, B., & Walsh, J. (2000). Win-win mentoring. *Nursing Management, 31* (1), 32–34.

Tannen, D. (1990). *You just do not understand: Women and men in conversation.* New York: William Morrow.

Tuohy, D. (2003). Student nurse-older person communication. *Nurse Education Today, 23* (1), 19–26.

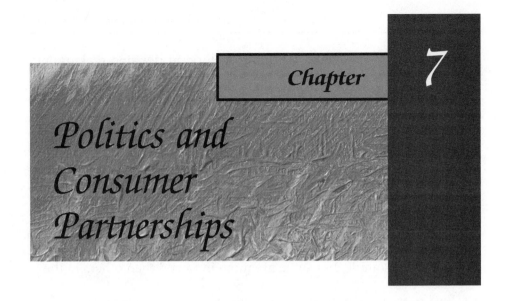

Chapter 7

Politics and Consumer Partnerships

Essential Concepts in Politics and Consumer Partnerships

The field of nursing is experiencing renewed interest because of a variety of factors, including the current nursing shortage, patient-to-staff ratio determinations in several states, and recent research illustrating that a higher quality of care is found where more registered nurses are employed. One component of this increased recognition concerning the role that nurses play in the delivery of quality care is through political awareness and activity by a variety of sources. The American Nurses Association (http://www.ana.org) offers a political voice representing the more than 2 million registered nurses in the United States.

Politics are found in every organization, regardless of its size or mission, and are generally considered to be the effective use of power to accomplish designated goals. Nurses cannot control the politics in their organization, but by increasing their political understanding and skills, they will improve their own power base and reach their goals and objectives. Learning political strategies is often a complex process for novice managers. Knowing whom to include in decision-making and information sharing is sometimes challenging. Strategies such as improving communication techniques, building a power base (both formal and informal), taking calculated risks in attempting to achieve new goals, developing personal alliances, and believing in yourself can go a long way toward making one politically savvy.

Politics and Their Effects on Health Care

- Politics affect every person in almost every aspect of their daily life.
- Stakeholders are those with a stake in a particular topic or issue. Everyone has an interest in the health care system of the United States, for example, but some are more involved than others in the policy-making process.
- Third-party payers, specifically health insurance companies, the government, and business, are also stakeholders who are increasingly political, especially when it comes to cost issues.
- Issues of diversity, including cultural, ethnic, gender, abilities, economic, social, and age issues, need to be considered as strategic components in the policy-making process. The rapidly aging population has the potential to affect health care delivery at every level, from preventative care to terminal care, with its significant political ramifications.

Nurse Involvement in the Political Process

- Although they are the largest health care provider group in the United States, nurses have not always successfully applied their power to the political arena. Efforts generally have centered on patient care services and issues of access policy. There is a significant need for nurses not only to be aware but also involved in policy development and implementation.
- To learn the political process, nurses can join their professional and specialty organizations and become involved with many policy-influencing activities. For example, the American Association of Nurse Anesthetists (http://www.aana.org), an effective practice organization, has a strong influence over legislation that affects the practice of nurse anesthetists in the United States.
- Nurses need to communicate both clearly and consistently what nursing is as a profession and what critical roles nurses play in assisting patients and their families with maintaining and achieving health.

- A strong and strategically political role for nurses is that of advocacy for their patients and their families.
- Because of sheer numbers—and with the positive view in which the public holds the profession of nursing—nurses hold significant voting power that can influence political outcomes.

Nurses and the New Consumer

- Because of increasingly available technologies, patients and their families are more informed about their health and illnesses than ever before. Contributing to the patients' knowledge base is the Internet and the media that discuss legal, ethical, political, economic, and social issues along with health-related concerns. Today, patients receive health information not only from their physician but also from nurses and other allied health practitioners as well as from neighbors and friends.
- To have credibility with the public, nurses need to demonstrate that they are both professional and competent, providing compassionate as well as quality manner.
- Nurses who work collaboratively with consumers can increase the potential for health care to be effective politically.

CASE SCENARIOS

Guided Case Scenario 7-1

You have relocated to a new state with an active state nurses association that is involved with nursing quality indicators at many of the hospitals. One day, you come into the break room and hear several of the more experienced nurses on the unit discussing the need for nurses to become more politically active because of the higher staffing ratios they encountered when first entering the profession more than 30 years ago. They are concerned that with the decreasing numbers of registered nurses and the increasing use of unlicensed assistive personnel (UAPs), patients are not getting the same quality of care that they used to receive. You are intrigued with their conversation. When you were in college, you were an active member of that state's student nurses association, working on a state task force for increasing the political awareness of student nurses.

Case Considerations

1. You ask the more seasoned nurses what you, as a staff nurse, can do to address this problem. Where would you start? What is the purpose of the state nurses association?
2. What can one do as an individual? What can be accomplished as a larger group?
3. What other political groups would be interested in joining with the nursing profession to alter the various aspects of health care delivery?
4. How does one join the state nurses association, and of what value is this?

Case Analysis

1. You ask the more seasoned nurses what you, as a staff nurse, can do to address this problem. Where would you start? What is the purpose of a state nurses association?

   You agree that many nurses together have a stronger voice than you do alone. One of the goals of a state nurses association is to be a voice for nurses in that state. As an example of such an association, the Virginia Nurses Association (http://www.virginianurses.com) ". . . promulgates standards of nursing practice, provides continuing education for nurses and influences public policy related to nursing practice and the consumer's health. The Association further believes that nurses are autonomous, prepared practitioners who are accountable for their practice and who are advocates for the consumer. [They] believe that nurses meet the health needs of the consumer through use of the nursing process and engagement in lifelong learning. The Association believes nursing is a self-regulated profession which engages in unified action and collaborates with others to meet the health care needs of consumers" (Virginia Nurses Association, 2002).

2. What can one do as an individual? What can be accomplished as a larger group?

   As an individual, one can certainly speak about personal opinions and become politically active to continue advocating both quality patient care and workplace issues that affect nurses. By joining recognized professional organizations, such as the state nurses association or one of the many specialty organizations, a nurse becomes part of a much larger voice. Larger groups often have lobbying powers, influencing those who are in position to change and enact legislation at the local, state, and national levels. As professionals, nurses have a responsibility to impact health care policy that both directly and indirectly affects the delivery of health care delivery.

3. What other political groups would be interested in joining with the nursing profession to alter the various aspects of health care delivery?

   Many groups are concerned with the delivery of costs of, access to, and quality of health care, as well as with health care policy and adequate preparation of health care professionals. As the population ages, the American Association of Retired Persons (http://www.aarp.org) becomes a stronger voice for policy changes, particularly regarding the rising health care costs that can greatly restrict an elder's budget. At the other end of the spectrum are consumer groups that focus on the health care and related policy of children and pregnant women. Ensuring that all women have access to adequate prenatal care decreases the chances of complications during childbirth and of premature babies, eventually decreasing the time of hospitalization and the resulting costs. Still other groups advocate for mental health issues, such as the Alzheimer's Association; are disease specific, such as the Leukemia Association; and focus on the political initiatives affecting health care access for the homeless. All would welcome the expertise and knowledge of a registered nurse who also believes in the goals of their organization.

4. How does one join a state nurses association, and of what value is this?

   As a registered nurse, it is easy for you to join a state nurses association. All states have a reduced rate for new graduates during the first year, so this is a wonderful oppor-tunity to join and become involved at a lower cost. Most, if not all, state associations also have a website; you could either print out an application and mail it in or complete the application on-line. By joining the state nurses association and, thereby, becoming a member of the larger American Nurses Association, one has a political avenue in which to voice opinions and to facilitate change at the local, regional, and national levels.

Case Scenario 7-2

The nursing shortage is not an unexpected phenomenon in the twenty-first century. Given that almost half the active registered nurses are scheduled to retire in the next decade, nursing educators and health care administrators alike acknowledge that this shortage has the potential to significantly impact health care regardless of the setting. This situation affects many different constituencies, including consumers of health care, patients, and even communities themselves as they provide health care services for their citizens.

Case Considerations

1. Many reasons are given for the current nursing shortage. What reasons are you aware of that have contributed to this issue?
2. What are some of the reasons that you were drawn to the nursing profession? Does it concern you that many of your colleagues will be retiring in the next decade? What could be the potential ramifications?
3. Many states are beginning to look at ways to attract more applicants into nursing schools or have established programs and developed policy for applicants and current students. Describe some of the initiatives you are aware of that address the issue of attracting more students into the nursing profession.
4. Identify some of the potential fallout from a decreasing pool of registered nurses. What are the political implications for hospitals and other providers of care? For third-party payers? For schools of higher education?
5. Certain populations, such as the elderly, those of minority cultures, and other vulnerable groups, are rapidly expanding in the United States. With a decreasing supply of nurses, what could the potential impact be on these populations and their health status?

Case Analysis

There is not one single reason why the nursing profession is declining in its numbers, but many factors are contributing to the shortage. When considering the possible impact of the decline in registered nurses, especially as our population in the United States continues to age as well as to develop more of a multicultural face, one needs to look beyond the usual places where nurses work.

Hospitals, clinics, and nursing homes are all affected when there is a shortage, but so are other areas, such as schools systems, colleges, and universities.

■ KEY POINTS

1. The number of students applying to nursing programs has been declining for the past several years. Only in the last year have baccalaureate programs seen an increase in applications. Some of the reasons for this increase include a sluggish economy, new loan-forgiveness programs for nursing students, health care systems providing scholarships, and hospitals realizing that to provide quality outcomes, registered nurses need to be at the patient's bedside providing care.
2. With the current nursing shortage, many states have become politically aware and involved with the education of nurses and are offering numerous incentives for students to enroll in a nursing program. Various policy makers have approved tuition reimbursements, loan-forgiveness programs, and other inducement programs (e.g., mortgage reductions). Hospital and health care lobbyists have spoken loudly about the nursing shortage and have asked that the states respond with these programs.
3. While the number of nurses as providers of care has declined, a significant shortage of nursing faculty has also developed. Although plenty of students may apply to fill openings in a nursing school, a shortage of faculty means that many of these slots cannot be filled.
4. An emphasis on developing future nursing faculty is just beginning. New or revised programs at the graduate level for nurse educators have appeared, as have many more opportunities regarding loan forgiveness for nursing faculty.
5. The changing face of the American population requires continuing education for nurses as they learn to care for increased numbers of patients who are elderly and from a multicultural background.

Reference

Virginia Nurses Association (2002). *Philosophy statement.* Retrieved October 10, 2002, from http://www.virginianurses.com

Suggested Readings

Buerhaus, P. I., Staiger, D. O., & Auerbach, D. I. (2000). Implications of an aging registered nurse workforce. *Journal of the American Medical Association, 283,* 2948–2954.

Davis, G. (2002). Why I would never consider not being a member of ANA. *South Carolina Nurse, 9* (2), 19.

Dobos, C. (2002). Why I won't even consider not belonging to SCNA-ANA. *South Carolina Nurse, 9* (1), 30.

Fagan, C. (1998). Nursing research and the erosion of care. *Nursing Outlook, 46* (6), 256–261.

Foley, M. (2000). ANA: Advocating for appropriate nurse staffing. *Imprint, 47* (5), 42.

Gebbie, K. M., Wakefield, M., & Kerfoot, K. (2000). Nursing and health policy. *Image: Journal of Nursing Scholarship, 32* (3), 307–314.

Griggith, J. (1999). *The well-managed health care organization.* Chicago: Health Administration Press.

Kramer, J. (1990). Trends to watch at the magnet hospitals. *Nursing, 90,* 67–74.

Mason, D., & Leavitt, J. K. (1999). *Policy and politics in nursing and health* care (3rd ed.). Philadelphia: W. B. Saunders.

Mason, D. J. (2003). It's all the rage: Disagreement—political or otherwise—can be healthy. *American Journal of Nursing, 103* (5), 11.

Meisenheimer, C. G. (1997). *Improving quality.* Gaithersburg, MD: Aspen Publishers.

Milstead, J. A. (1999). *Health policy & politics: A nurse's guide.* Gaithersburg, MD: Aspen Publishers.

Shui, L., & Singh, D. A. (2001). *Delivering health care in America* (2nd ed.). Gaithersburg, MD: Aspen Publishers.

Sultz, H. A., & Young, K. M. (1999). *Health care USA* (2nd ed.). Gaithersburg, MD: Aspen Publishers.

Wieck, K. L. (2003). President's notes: Power, policy and politics. *Texas Nursing, 7* (1), 8.

Wolper, L. (1999). *Health care administration planning, implementing and managing organized delivery systems* (3rd ed.). Gaithersburg, MD: Aspen Publishers.

Planning Care

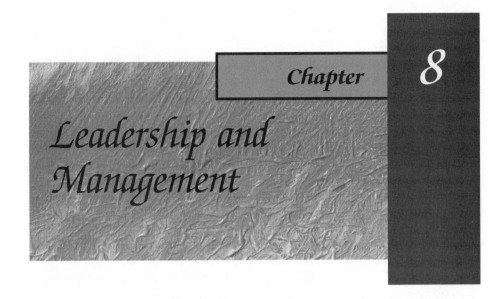

Chapter *8*

Leadership and Management

Essential Concepts in Leadership and Management

Theories abound regarding the development and roles of both leaders and managers in today's business environment. Nurse managers need a solid foundation in both management and leadership to function effectively within a changing health care setting, where issues of resource management, personnel coaching, and managing change require up-to-date information.

Management theory has developed over the last century, and certain tenets of the original management process are still being applied today. Management focuses on the daily operations of a given setting, with staffing, budgeting, counseling, and discipline being a few examples of these functions. What has changed in management theory today is the increasing focus on the employee and his or her motivational level, satisfaction with the work and the work environment, and relationship with both managers and subordinates. Leadership, or the ability to move a group toward a common goal, is widely applied in a variety of settings and situations, with the objective being an effective leader in a changing work environment.

Nurses are both managers and leaders on a daily basis, regardless of position. Staff nurses manage and coordinate the nursing care of those patients under their supervision, and they may simultaneously be leading a team of care providers. Likewise, nurse managers also need the skills sets of both management and leadership, because different situations require diverse leadership styles and management decisions.

Management and the Management Process

- Management functions center on coordinating tasks, accomplishments, and allocation of resources.
- Fayol (1916/1949) identifies the four functions of management: planning, organizing, coordinating, and controlling.
- Gulick and Urwick (1937) further identify seven principles of the management process: planning, organizing, staffing, directing, coordinating, reporting, and budgeting.

Key Management Theories

- Taylor (1911) developed the Scientific Management Theory, which focused on increasing productivity based on the systematic investigation of processes.
- Weber (1922/1946) is known for his Bureaucratic Theory, which outlines the bureaucratic organization's need for superior-subordinate relationships with clear communication patterns, formal structures, and chain of command.
- In the Hawthorne Studies conducted in 1930, Mayo (1933) discovered that employees increased their productivity when they were being observed by others. The Hawthorne effect occurs when someone's behavior is altered because of being studied.

Motivational Theories

- Maslow (1970) offered the Hierarchy of Needs Theory (Figure 8-1), which suggests that a person's basic needs must be fulfilled before he or she can be motivated to satisfy someone else's need.
- Herzberg (1968) developed the Two-Factor Theory of motivation. He believed that certain factors, or motivators, lead to job satisfaction; these include the work itself, achievement, responsibility, recognition, and the possibility for growth and advancement. Other factors, called hygiene factors, contribute to job dissatisfaction;

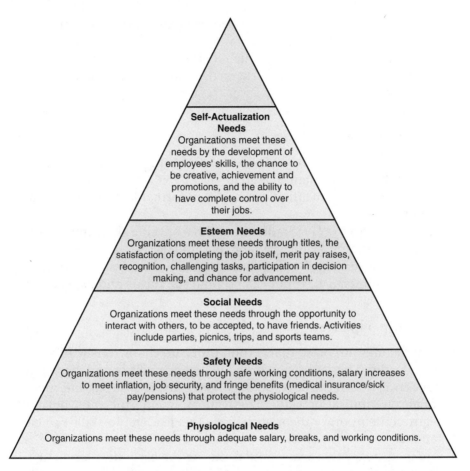

Figure 8-1   How Organizations Motivate with the Hierarchy of Needs
Theory. From Lussier, R. N., & Achua, C. F. (2001). *Leader-
ship: Theory, application, skill building* (p. 81). Cincinnati,
OH: South-Western College.

when present, they lead to a decreased motivational level. These
hygiene factors are salary, supervision, status in the company,
company policies, and job security. Even one's personal life has
influence over job dissatisfaction. Overall, Herzberg believed that
work itself can be the motivation and that an employee has an
internal drive to succeed.

• McGregor (1960) contributed the Theory X and Theory Y dichotomy,
which examines what motivates people to be actively involved at
work. Theory X managers believe that most people are at work
simply to obtain their paycheck and must be constantly supervised.

Theory Y managers believe that people enjoy work and want to contribute, regardless of the rewards.
- Theory Z was developed by Ouchi (1981). It focuses on the involvement and participation of workers, especially in developing quality products.

Leadership Characteristics

- Leadership is the ability to influence others to perform and work toward the achievement of a goal.
- Leaders in an organization can be either formal leaders or informal leaders.
- Bennis and Nanus (1985) identified three specific characteristics of leaders: a guiding vision, passion, and integrity.
- Other traits attributed to many leaders include a desire to lead, honesty, enthusiasm, support, and high standards and expectations.

Leadership Theories

- Trait theories advocate that certain traits are characteristic of a great leader. These traits include intelligence, self-confidence, independence, nonconformity, personal integrity, and strong interpersonal communication skills. These are all wonderful traits, but many contemporary theorists believe that leadership skills can be taught.
- Another theory that was popular during the early development of leadership studies is the Great Man Theory, which promotes the notion that a leader is born with certain innate abilities and leads those who are not born to be leaders but, rather, are born to be led. This theory is no longer popular.
- The behavioral approach to leadership theory identifies three leadership styles: autocratic, democratic, and laissez-faire. In this theory, a leader may use all three, depending on the situation.
- Two basic leadership behaviors are employee-centered leadership, in which the leader is focused on developing others and on high-performance goals, and job-centered leadership, which does not emphasize the human needs aspect of the employees (Lewin, 1939).
- Fielder (1967) developed the Contingency Theory, which states that leadership behavior depends on the personality of the leader and on each particular situation. In this theory, no one leader is optimal in all settings. Leader-member relations, task structure, and position power are all factors in the effectiveness of a leader.

- The Situational Theory of Hersey and Blanchard (2000) looks not only at a leader's effectiveness but also includes the follower's readiness, which is also known as maturity.
- In the Path-Goal Theory of House (1971), the leader makes the path easier for the follower by using the appropriate behavior (e.g., directive, supportive, participative, or achievement-oriented).
- Servant leadership (Greenleaf, 1998) involves leading others through respect, trust, and collaboration while practicing active listening skills.

Transactional Versus Transformational Leadership

- In the Transactional Leadership Theory of Burns (1978), the leader is mostly concerned with daily operations and is not as involved with people development. Instead, the leader sets strategic goals and deals with risk-taking initiatives.
- The transformational leader strives to empower others and to motivate followers by articulating his or her vision and behaving as an agent of change. Transformational leaders can be anyone in the organization, regardless of the position held.

CASE SCENARIOS

Guided Case Scenario 8-1

Hannah is the senior evening staff registered nurse (RN) and has worked on your floor for the last 10 years. Her patient care is certainly adequate, but her interpersonal behavior is becoming increasingly more difficult for her coworkers to deal with. She throws charts around the unit, gives curt answers to questions, and appears generally unhappy. She tells the staff that they are lazy and require her close supervision because of their lack of accountability and responsibility.

You have been hired, from the outside, as the new evening charge nurse. You already informally counseled Hannah a month ago about her behavior. It was an uncomfortable situation to discuss with her, but her coworkers had insisted that something be done. In fact, the previous charge nurse became so frustrated with Hannah's "my way or no way" behavior that she transferred to another floor.

Now, Hannah is beginning to intimidate the three newly hired graduate nurses. They have come to you requesting a transfer to another floor, saying that Hannah insists on knowing what they are doing at all times and that Hannah claims there is only one right way to do things. They also feel that Hannah does not trust them and insists on checking everything they do.

Case Considerations

1. Which management theory and/or theorist does Hannah illustrate, and why?
2. Which management theory and/or theorist may be more desirable to apply to this situation, and why?
3. How would you, as the manager of this shift, help to develop Hannah's management and supervisory skills, particularly in the area of people skills?
4. What are some more desirable leadership traits to develop in Hannah?

Case Analysis

1. Which management theory and/or theorist does Hannah illustrate, and why?

   Hannah clearly exhibits the Theory X management style of McGregor (1960). Theory X managers assume they need to keep on top of their employees at all times, because the employees are irresponsible and try to get out of as much work as possible. A manager such as Hannah is difficult to work with. These managers do not necessarily trust their employees and feel that they have to provide the extrinsic motivation, because they believe that employees have no intrinsic motivation to perform well and do their best.

   Another perspective on Hannah's management style is gained by applying the work of Lewin (1939) on leadership style. Of the three styles of leadership—autocratic, democratic, and laissez-faire—the one that most exemplifies Hannah's management style is autocratic. An autocratic leader makes most of the decisions without consulting his or her subordinates, and this type of leader uses power to control the environment rather than seeking input from the employees.

2. Which management theory and/or theorist may be more desirable to apply to this situation, and why?

   McGregor (1960) did not view his Theory X and Theory Y as being polar opposites. Many others do, however, because the characteristics are quite different. One is not seen as being inherently more desirable than the other, but most would agree that Theory Y is the preferred management perspective. Theory Y managers believe that employees like their work, want to be at work, and act in a responsible, self-directed manner, needing little assistance and supervision from the manager. It is highly unlikely, however, that any manager has pure Theory X or pure Theory Y assumptions about their employees. Most tend to fall somewhere on a continuum based on the situation, the employees, and the manager.

3. How would you, as the manager of this shift, help to develop Hannah's management and supervisory skills, particularly in the area of people skills?

One of the first things to do is sit with Hannah and obtain her perspective on her own management style. Some people truly do not know how they appear to others, and they are genuinely surprised when confronted. If she appears unhappy and is throwing things and speaking curtly, you need to find out if this is new behavior or a continuation of something that has been going on many years without anyone addressing it. Something may be happening in Hannah's personal life that is affecting her at work. Although this is not an excuse, it sometimes helps to understand what some of an employee's issues are, and you can perhaps offer suggestions for assisting Hannah.

As Hannah's manager, you should try to find out why she treats her coworkers poorly and, at times, does not trust their abilities or decisions. Maybe Hannah would benefit from a course on developing supervisory skills, or an opportunity may exist for some continuing education on leadership topics. Most of all, Hannah needs to develop an awareness of how she appears to others and how to treat her coworkers with more respect and trust—two characteristics that are difficult to teach. Of concern are the staff nurses who would rather transfer to another unit than work with Hannah, who needs to know how her behavior is affecting staff morale, teamwork, and eventually, retention of nurses.

4. What are some more desirable leadership traits to develop in Hannah?

Ultimately, it would be wonderful if Hannah would develop empathy and understanding toward her coworkers; however, you will take a pleasant demeanor toward them. You are seeking someone who wants to be at work and who believes that others want to be there as well. She may do well with some basic supervisory skill development, coaching, and mentoring from a more experienced leader on the unit. As the manager, it is important to emphasize that Hannah's clinical skills are satisfactory and are not the focus of the discussion, which is about her interpersonal skills.

Case Scenario 8-2

One of your assignments in class is to discuss the differences between managers and leaders. Some in your class believe that leaders are born with leadership qualities, but others argue that leaders are taught these qualities. All, however, agree that you can teach most people how to be effective managers.

Case Considerations

1. Are most leaders born with leadership tendencies, or can leaders be taught these skills?
2. What are the differences between managers and leaders? Which of their qualities are similar? Which of their qualities are different?
3. Who comes to mind when someone asks you to think of a great leader? How about a great manager? Which person is harder to find as an example, and why?
4. Think of someone who you believe had great management and leadership skills and qualities. What were those skills and qualities, and how did they acquire them?
5. Think of someone who you believe had poor management and leadership characteristics. Describe some of these characteristics and how they affected the people being supervised. What could have been improved in this person's skills?

Case Analysis

Outstanding management and leadership characteristics are skills that not everyone possesses in limitless amounts, regardless of the situation or of those who are being supervised. Both are skill sets that contain learned behaviors, and both require some inherent understanding that cannot be taught from a book or even from direct experience.

■ *KEY POINTS*

1. Be sure to differentiate between management and leadership skills and characteristics. One can be a great leader yet be a little short on management qualities, and vice versa.
2. Sometimes, the best way to learn how to be an effective leader and manager is to have a mentor or coach who assists you in developing these skills. Name someone you know who would be a great mentor.
3. People with poor leadership and management styles often have difficulty working effectively with their staff and others. A large component of management and leadership capability is effective people skills and, above all, the ability to communicate to a variety of people in a variety of settings and in ways that are determined by the situation.

References

Bennis, W., & Nannus, B. (1985). *Leaders: The strategies for taking charge.* New York: Harper & Row.

Burns, J. M. (1978). *Leadership.* New York: Harper & Row.

Fayol, H. (1916/1949). (C. Storrs, Trans.). *General and industrial management.* London: Pitman.

Fielder, F. (1967). *A theory of leadership effectiveness.* New York: McGraw-Hill.

Greenleaf, R. K. (1998). *The power of servant leadership.* San Francisco: Berrett-Koehler.

Gulick, L., & Urwick, L. (Eds.). (1937). *Papers on the science of administration.* New York: Institute of Public Administration.

Hersey, P., & Blanchard, K. (2000). *Management of organizational behavior* (8th ed.). Englewood Cliffs, NJ: Prentice Hall.

Herzberg, F. (1968). One more time: How do you motivate employees? *Harvard Business Review,* (January/February), 53–62.

House, R. H. (1971). A path-goal theory of leader effectiveness. *Administration Science Quarterly, 16,* 321–338.

Lewin, K. (1939). Field theory and experiment in social psychology: Concepts and methods. *Journal of Sociology, 44,* 868–896.

Maslow, A. (1970). *Motivation and personality* (2nd ed.). New York: Harper & Row.

Mayo, E. (1933). *The human problems of an industrial civilization.* New York: Macmillan.

McGregor, D. (1960). *The human side of enterprise.* New York: McGraw-Hill.

Ouchi, W. (1981). *Theory Z: How American business can meet the Japanese challenge.* Reading, MA: Addison-Wesley.

Taylor, F. (1911). *Principles of scientific management.* New York: Harper & Row.

Weber, M. (1922/1946). (H. H. Gerth & C. W. Mills, Trans.). *Max Weber: Essays in sociology.* London: Oxford University Press.

Suggested Readings

Antrobus, S., & Kitson, A. (1999). Nursing leadership: Influencing and shaping health policy and nursing practice. *Journal of Advanced Nursing, 29,* 746–753.

Bass, B. (1980). *Bass and Stodgill's handbook of leadership.* New York: Free Press.

Benefield, L. E., Clifford, J., Cos, S., Hagenow, N. R., Hastings, C., & Kobs, A. (2000). Nursing leaders predict top trends for 2000. *Nursing Management, 31* (1), 21–23.

Daft., R. L., & Marcic, D. (2001). *Understanding management* (3rd ed.). Philadelphia: Harcourt College.

Drucker, P. (1999). *Management challenges for the 21st century.* New York: Harper Business.

Faugier, J., & Woolnough, H. (2001). Breaking the male mold: A new approach to leadership. *Mental Health Practice, 4* (9), 6–8.

Griggith, J. (1999). *The well-managed health care organization.* Chicago: Health Administration Press.

Gurian, M. (2001). *Boys and girls learn differently.* San Francisco: Jossey-Bass.

Horton-Deutsch, S. L., & Mohr, W. K. (2001). The fading of nursing leadership. *Nursing Outlook, 49,* 121–126.

Kerfoot, K. (2003). On leadership. Creating your own leadership brand. *MED-SURG Nursing, 12* (2), 132–134.

Kotter, J. (1990). What leaders really do. *Harvard Business Review, 68,* 104.

Kramer, J. (1990). Trends to watch at the magnet hospitals. *Nursing, 90* (June), 67–74.

Krau, S. D. (2002). Leadership circle. Men in nursing: A different voice and a different brain. *SCI Nursing, 19* (3), 138–141.

Marquis, B. L., & Huston, C. J. (2000). *Leadership roles and management functions* (3rd ed.). Philadelphia: J. B. Lippincott.

McGee-Cooper, A., & Looper, G. (2001). *The essentials of servant leadership: Principles in practice.* Waltham, MA: Pegasus Communications.

Porter-O'Grady, T. (1999). Quantum leadership: New roles for a new age. *Journal of Nursing Administration, 29* (10), 37–42.

Sofarelli, M., & Brown, R. (1998). The need for nursing leadership in uncertain times. *Journal of Nursing Management, 6* (4), 201–207.

Valentine, S. O. (2002). Nursing leadership and the new nurse. *Journal for Undergraduate Nursing Scholarship, 4* (1), 4–8.

Ward, K. (2002). A vision for tomorrow: Transformational nursing leaders. *Nursing Outlook, 50* (3): 121–126.

Williams, D. (2002). Looking for a few good men. *Minority Nurse,* 22–27.

Wolper, L. (1999). *Health care administration planning, implementing and managing organized delivery systems* (3rd ed.). Gaithersburg, MD: Aspen Publishers.

Yukl, G. (2002). *Leadership in organizations* (4th ed.). Upper Saddle River, NJ: Prentice Hall.

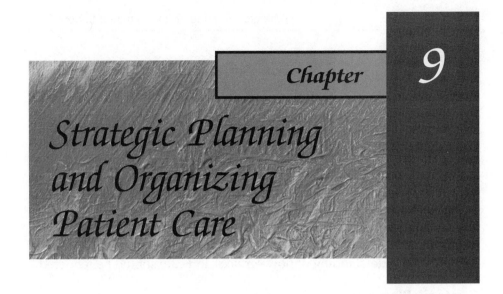

Chapter 9

Strategic Planning and Organizing Patient Care

Essential Concepts in Strategic Planning and Organizing Patient Care

An effective planning process is crucial to the success of any organization. In planning, many alternatives are examined, in a proactive manner, for their impact on the organization. Therefore, many possibilities are reviewed for their potential to achieve the desired results and their congruence with the mission of the organization. Every health care organization has a specific mission and philosophy that grow out of their expressed values and beliefs. A strategic plan needs to be consistent and congruent with the mission so that the organization does not stray from its primary reason for existence.

Health care organizations have many differing structures, which enables them to carry out their mission, philosophy, and strategic plan efficiently. Organizations can be structured in a matrix or hierarchical manner, and the power base can be decentralized or centralized. Regardless of the structure, well-communicated reporting relationships are needed to ensure a clearly defined division of labor.

Mission

- A mission is the reason that an organization exists and is defined by the organization's purpose statement. The mission statement influences the organization in everything that it is, because it guides the development of the philosophy, goals, and objectives. Beliefs and values drive the development of the mission statement.

Philosophy

- An organization's philosophy often reflects its values and beliefs and is more in-depth than the mission statement. The mission and philosophy of an organization should be consistent and give both employees and clients an understanding of how services and care should be rendered.

Strategic Planning

- Strategic planning is the process of setting goals and objectives for an organization, with an identified period for accomplishment. The steps in strategic planning are summarized in Table 9-1.
- A strategic plan emerges when an organization analyzes the current environmental situation and arrives at goals to achieve the desired change. The ultimate goal of a dynamic strategic plan is to provide a "road map" for the planning process, with the goal of being organizational growth and improvement.
- The first step in the strategic planning process begins with an organizational assessment, which is also called an environmental analysis or scan.

Table 9-1   Summary of Steps in Strategic Planning

1. Perform an environmental assessment.
2. Conduct a stakeholder analysis.
3. Review the literature for evidence and best practices.
4. Determine congruence with the organizational mission.
5. Identify the planning goals and objectives.
6. Estimate the resources required for the plan.
7. Prioritize according to available resources.
8. Identify timelines and responsibilities.
9. Develop a marketing plan.
10. Write and communicate the business or strategic plan.
11. Evaluate.

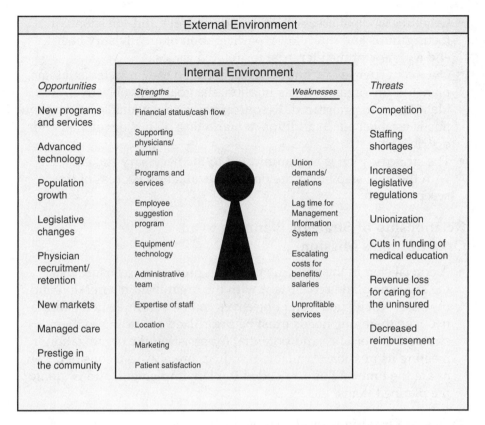

Figure 9-1   Key to Success in Strategic Planning: SWOT Analysis.

- The second step facilitates the environmental assessment and is a SWOT (strengths, weaknesses, opportunities, and threats) analysis (Figure 9-1). The SWOT analysis is often used during the initial brainstorming sessions, in which everybody involved with the strategic planning process offers opinions of the internal strengths and weaknesses of the organization and the opportunities and threats of the external environment.
- During the third step, many stakeholders are surveyed regarding their opinions of the organization's needs. A stakeholder is someone, whether internal or external to the organization, who has a vested interest in the organization and its services. It is critical to involve as many stakeholders as possible during the assessment phase, not only because they can offer different perspectives but also to encourage a sense of ownership of the resulting findings.

- Other methods of assessment include surveys and questionnaires, focus groups and interviews, participation of an advisory board, and a review of the literature for related issues.
- Once congruence is acknowledged between the projected strategic plan and the organization's mission, the goals and objectives are identified and prioritized. Resources are made available, and a time-line is established. In addition, a marketing plan is developed and distributed.
- The strategic plan is communicated to the necessary stakeholders, with the final step being the ongoing evaluation process of the accepted plan.

Relationship of Strategic Planning to an Organization's Mission

- A crucial step in the strategic planning process is to ensure that the strategic plan is consistent with the organization's mission and purpose. Not all goals and objectives can be accomplished simultaneously; therefore, needs must be prioritized according to their strategic importance and potential for assisting the organization in meeting its mission. Available resources are always a consideration, as are the time and effort needed to plan, implement, and evaluate the planned items.

Types of Organizational Structures

- In a centralized organization, much of the decision-making occurs at the top administrative level. In contrast, a decentralized organization makes decisions throughout the ranks and seeks input from the different managerial levels.
- Reporting relationships can be illustrated on an organizational chart, which has a place for many of the positions within an organization. When viewing an organizational chart, one can easily identify reporting mechanisms and the division of labor, which generally is based either on geographic area or on type of service or product area.

CASE SCENARIOS

Guided Case Scenario 9-1

One of the fastest-growing service lines in your hospital is cardiac services. Because your hospital does not have a dedicated cardiac floor, telemetry unit, or intensive care unit, cardiac patients are admitted to any open bed. You manage a 10-bed step-down unit and a 40-bed medical-surgical unit. You have been the manager for almost 8 years. Before you became the nurse manager at this hospital, you worked in a nearby city as the day charge nurse in the coronary care unit.

The Chief Nursing Officer (CNO) asks you to join her in a planning meeting with other administrators of the health care system. During the meeting, hospital expansion soon becomes a topic of the discussion, as does the lack of available beds because of a consistently high census year-round. The Chief Executive Officer (CEO) turns to the CNO and asks what area she would recommend capitalizing on during the next few years because of high patient growth and community demand. The CNO states that she believes cardiac care will continue to increase for numerous reasons, including increased census, new physician recruitment in this area, an aging population, and other factors. All the other administrators agree, and the CEO asks the CNO to devise a strategic plan centering on expansion of the cardiac service line.

Case Considerations

1. Describe strategic planning.
2. What comprises the strategic planning process?
3. Where does one begin the strategic planning process with this project?
4. What type of timeline can one anticipate for this project?
5. Who should be involved with this cardiac project, and why? Who are the stakeholders, both in the hospital and in the community?
6. Identify some of the issues to be included in the strategic plan.
7. Tentatively outline the SWOT process and some of the potential considerations for each area.

Case Analysis

1. Describe strategic planning.

   Strategic planning is the concerted effort by an organization to plan the direction of the organization, taking into account its mission, philosophy, values, and interest from stakeholders. It is a proactive process, whereby designated parties contribute to this cyclic course of action, mapping out future goals and strategies.

2. What comprises the strategic planning process?

    The strategic planning process is comprised of an assessment phase, a planning phase, an implementation phase, and an evaluation phase (after the plan has been initiated). Different phases take varying times to accomplish and often are dependent on the stakeholders involved and the information available.

3. Where does one begin the strategic planning process with this project?

    The most important phase of the strategic planning process and possibly the one that takes the most time to complete, is the assessment phase. Why is this phase so essential and fundamental to an effective strategic plan? The assessment phase often involves the largest number of people and factors, both inside the organization (e.g., employees, physicians, and patients) and outside the organization (e.g., community needs as well as social, economic, and other factors).

    To initiate the assessment phase, one could begin with an environmental assessment that examines the broader setting in which the organization is situated. What are the influencing factors that mold how health care is delivered? Are special interest groups involved? What are the largest product lines? Which area of patient care has the greatest potential for growth? Which area of patient care is decreasing in numbers? What is the market share for certain products and services, and who else in the surrounding region offers these services? What are the reimbursement schedules of these desired services, and does a budget exist for them?

    A SWOT analysis can then be performed to assess the organization's strengths, weaknesses, opportunities, and threats. A SWOT analysis is often a great exercise for an organization, because it involves brainstorming early during the process, allowing a free flow and study of the organization's strengths, weaknesses, opportunities, and threats.

    Another step in the assessment phase is to perform a community and stakeholder assessment. This type of assessment can take several formats, including surveys and questionnaires, focus groups and interviews, and advice from an advisory board. In addition, a review of current literature is recommended to see if similar programs exist and what their outcomes have been.

4. What type of timeline can one anticipate for this project?

To accurately project a timeline for the development and initiation of a strategic plan, you need to have some information at the beginning. First, what is the depth of the projected project? Does it involve the development of a new product line or service or construction of a new building? These types of projects may take longer than simply "tweaking" an existing program. Does the new service or program involve the hiring and training of staff? Depending on the region of the country and the specialization, recruitment of staff may take some time to implement. Strategic plans are often performed every 2 or 3 years, with reviews occurring in-between or when a need arises for an additional service or project.

5. Who should be involved with this cardiac project, and why? Who are the stakeholders, both in the hospital and in the community?

The first step is to identify all the appropriate stakeholders, both internal and external to the organization. You could begin by identifying the cardiac physicians and referring physicians, then interviewing key members regarding their impressions. Do they see a need for an expansion of cardiac care? What would they like to see as far as services and programs?

After interviewing the physicians, nurses and the allied health professionals need to be interviewed for their opinions and viewpoints. How will the expansion of a cardiac service line affect them? Will increased staffing and education be needed? Where will you find new or additional staff? Who will be responsible for training them?

A look at the community, especially a review of the demographics and other socioeconomic indicators regarding your future patients, is helpful at this stage. It is also critical to examine what services are already available from competing health care systems to ensure that a need for expanding your services truly exists. After all, if the other health care systems all offer the same services and they are not seeing growth, is this a service that your organization really wants to initiate, or can the money, time, and energy be better placed elsewhere?

6. Identify some of the issues to be included in the strategic plan.

Before beginning any large-scale project and, perhaps, while simultaneously performing the assessment phase, it is crucial to identify the desired patient and organizational outcomes for initiating an expansion of cardiac care. To know where you are going with a project, you need to have clearly defined goals with defined outcomes.

Another issue is that of financing. Even if you come up with the most wonderful plan, there will be no way to complete the project if adequate funding is not available. Be sure to resolve this issue before actually initiating the project.

Timing is crucial. Many projects need the approval of state and local agencies, so deadlines in the application process may need to be met. Is there a specific time by which the project needs to be initiated or completed to secure and maintain a funding source?

7. Tentatively outline the SWOT process and some of the potential considerations for each area.

Strengths: Look to the internal and external strengths of the organization and of those that would be contributing to the project. Be sure to include issues of personnel, funding sources, profit potential, technology, marketing, location, building availability, space, physician support, community support, legislative opportunities, and the desire of the organization to take on the project.

Weaknesses: Review the internal and external weaknesses of the organization and of those that would be contributing to the project. Are there issues with any of the above-mentioned topics?

Opportunities: With the opportunity section, one is seeking to advance health care delivery in the defined area. Is there new legislation that enables the initiation of the new project? Are there new markets, new technology, opportunity for increased reimbursement and revenue, enhanced recruitment efforts, and potential for increased prestige in the community? Is there a service gap from the other health care systems that would benefit the community?

Threats: Threats are the opposite of opportunities. One needs to examine closely all the above-mentioned topics for any downside to the potential program or project.

Case Scenario 9-2

After taking this class, you realize your life could use a little strategic planning. You are graduating next semester, and you are unsure of what you want to do, where you want to live, and what direction your life will take without the regimen of college.

Case Considerations

1. How can you apply the fundamentals of strategic planning to your life planning?
2. What are the steps that you will take?
3. What are your goals in performing a strategic plan for after graduation?

Case Analysis

Strategic planning is not just for organizational planning. Strategic planning can be undertaken for almost any project with which you are involved. The rudiments of this type of planning involve a structured process that can be applied consistently, regardless of setting, program, or project.

■ KEY POINTS

1. Begin your strategic plan with a SWOT analysis. What are your strengths in terms of experiences, both in and out of school? Who can assist you in a new job? Is one location more favorable than others? Will friends or family influence your decision? For weaknesses, look again to the above-mentioned topics. Is a move to another location or city a positive or a negative? Do you have direct experiences in one clinical area, or are you seeking a career in something brand new? Opportunities and threats can be viewed in the same manner. You can see new opportunities as doors opening up for you, or they can be intimidating. You need to understand yourself well to distinguish those situations that promise growth and challenges from those situations that could immobilize you from anxiety.
2. Before you make any decisions, be sure to understand your goals. Goals do not have to be long term (e.g., for the next 5 years), but they should reach far enough into the future to enable you to put together a reasonable plan of action. If you want to return to graduate school in 2 years so that you can become a nurse anesthetist, you need to look for a job opportunity that will give you the necessary experiences.

Suggested Readings

Bass, B. (1980). *Bass and Stodgill's handbook of leadership.* New York: Free Press.

Bennis, W., & Nannus, B. (1985). *Leaders: The strategies for taking charge.* New York: Harper & Row.

Burns, J. M. (1978). *Leadership.* New York: Harper & Row.

Daft., R. L., & Marcic, D. (2001). *Understanding management* (3rd ed.). Philadelphia: Harcourt College.

Drenkard, K. (2002). Invest the time to develop a "business plan." *Patient Care Staffing Report, 2* (1), 6–7.

Ecord, J. S. (2003). Critical connections. Nursing's agenda for the future. *Advances in Neonatal Care, 3* (1), 2.

Gessner, T. L. (1998). In J. A. Dienemann (Ed.), *Nursing administration: Managing patient care* (2nd ed., pp. 359–378). Stamford, CA: Appleton & Lange.

Griggith, J. (1999). *The well-managed health care organization.* Chicago: Health Administration Press.

Hayes, L. (2002). A primary care leadership program. *Primary Health Care, 12* (10), 22–25.

Levi, P. (1999). Sustainability of healthcare environments. *Image: Journal of Nursing Scholarship, 31* (4), 395–398.

Marquis, B. L., & Huston, C. J. (2000). *Leadership roles and management functions* (3rd ed.). Philadelphia: J. B. Lippincott.

McNichol, E. (2002). Thinking outside the box. *Nursing Management, 9* (4), 20–22.

Prescott, P. (2000). The enigmatic nursing workforce. *Journal of Nursing Administration, 30* (2), 59–65.

Sheetz, A. Z. (2002). Developing a strategic plan for school health services in Massachusetts. *Journal of School Health, 72* (7), 278–281.

Shortell, S., & Kaluzny, A. (2000). *Health care management: Organization design and behavior* (4th ed.). Clifton Park, NY: Delmar Learning.

Wolf, G. A. (2000). Vision 2000—The transformation of professional practice. *Nursing Administration Quarterly, 24* (2), 45–51.

Wolper, L. (1999). *Health care administration planning, implementing and managing organized delivery systems* (3rd ed.). Gaithersburg, MD: Aspen Publishers.

Yukl, G. (1998). *Leadership in organizations* (4th ed.). Upper Saddle River, NJ: Prentice Hall.

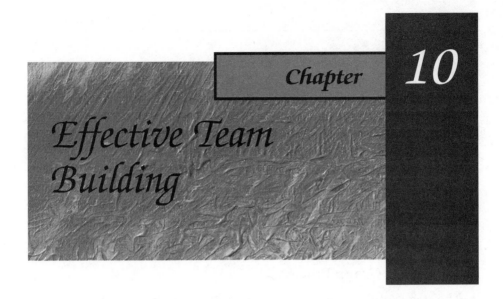

Chapter *10*

Effective Team Building

Essential Concepts of Team Building

Health care professionals do not work in isolation. All positions require some element of teamwork, and all require working interdependently at times as well as independently. It is essential that managers and leaders of nursing teams be aware that successful teams do not simply happen. Many times, successful teams are coached and mentored, teaching team members about the ideals that bring people together for a common purpose and goal. In this chapter, team roles are defined, and the stages of team development are identified. The team leader hopes that all members of the team will be useful and contribute to the overall goal, but in reality, teams often include dysfunctional members who hinder any progress from being made, no matter how small or insignificant. It takes a skilled team leader to move team members past any issues to reach the goals set at the beginning of the process.

Defining Teams and Committees

- Teams consist of a group of people with a common purpose and common performance goals. Each team member needs to contribute to the overall goal to have a successful team outcome.
- An interdisciplinary team is composed of members with a variety of expertise, both clinical and nonclinical, who meet for a common purpose.
- A committee is a work group with a specific task or goal to accomplish. An ad hoc committee is temporary and is formed for a specific purpose, time frame, or short-term goal. Some organizations will call an ad hoc committee a task force.

Stages of the Group Process

- The stages of the group process are outlined in Figure 10-1.
- In the forming phase, expectations, boundaries, and interactions are initiated with the new group members. What the team will hope to accomplish and how the group is to proceed toward that goal are curiosities to everyone at this point.
- The storming phase is the uncomfortable phase. Group members feel freer in their thoughts and conversations. Conflict and tension are hallmarks of the this phase.
- Norming occurs when equilibrium is again achieved within the group. In this stage, positive productivity begins.
- The performing phase is the most enjoyable phase. Generally, everyone agrees, and great progress is made toward accomplishing the stated vision and goals.
- The adjourning phase is the final stage of the group process. In this stage, group members evaluate their progress toward meeting the

Forming	Storming	Norming	Performing	Adjourning
• Expectations	• Tension	• Positioning	• Actual work	• Closure
• Interactions	• Conflict	• Goal setting	• Relationships	• Evaluation
• Boundary formation	• Confrontation	• Cohesiveness	• Group maturity	• Outcomes review

Figure 10-1   Stages of the Group Process. Based on Tuckman and Jensen (1977) and Lacoursier (1980).

expected goals and objectives. Closure needs to occur during this phase.

Key Concepts of Effective Teams

- The team has a clearly stated purpose or vision and an idea of what needs to be accomplished and by when.
- A clear assessment of the individual team members is made to identify the strengths and weaknesses of the group as a whole. Members are added or deleted based on the assessment results.
- A clear communication pattern is in place to ensure that information is disseminated both quickly and accurately to the team members and other stakeholders.
- The team leader encourages active participation by all team members, looking for their strengths in what they can contribute.

Creating an Environment Conducive to Team Building

- Closely review the environment in which the team meets to ensure that everyone's voice is heard.
- Make resources readily available when needed to the team, such as meeting space, audiovisual equipment, and secretarial support.
- Ensure that the administrators who formed the team and want it maintained are supportive of the team's efforts and goals, regardless of the results.
- Create a reward or recognition system for the team members as progress is made toward the established goal. People like to see themselves as well as others recognized for their achievements.
- Meetings should be productive, with noticeable results at their completion.

CASE SCENARIOS

Guided Case Study 10-1

You are a staff nurse on a 40-bed orthopedic floor. You thoroughly enjoy your role, but you wish that there were more opportunities for career growth. The Chief Nurse Executive overheard you making this comment to the charge nurse and has asked you to be the team leader of an already-established task force on falls that, frankly, has not really been effective. You are thrilled with the opportunity but also are a little nervous about being the team leader. Some of the current issues that the team needs to deal with include: 1) the increase in the incidence of falls, particularly in those occurring postoperatively on the medical-surgical floors; 2) the lack of team participation by the assigned team members; 3) a feeling by those both on and off the team that this task force is "just another thing to do during a busy day"; and 4) the lack of progress (nonproductivity) of the team.

During your first meeting as team leader, only 6 of the 20 members attend, and several of them are late. Watching the interactions between the staff, you begin to wonder if this group of professionals, because of all the differences in personalities and communication styles, can ever be effective in making decisions about the task of decreasing falls in the hospital. No one really even had an idea of what needed to be discussed at this meeting, so the first 20 minutes were spent talking about some of the previous night's staffing issues.

You note the different personalities around the table. Jamie is a new graduate nurse and volunteers for everything that needs to be done so that he will be liked. Angela is the detailer, often asking everyone to repeat what he or she said so that she can get more information on the topic. Samantha is the passive one and just looks annoyed at having to be there. You notice that Samantha was doing some of her patient charting while in the meeting. Annabelle attempts to keep the group on track, but with her soft-spoken voice, she is not well heard. Finally, Beth, no matter what anyone says, is critical and comes up with a reason why it will not work. Two hours later, you leave the meeting frustrated and doubting your ability to pull the team together.

Case Considerations

1. As the newly assigned team leader, do you feel challenged or overwhelmed?
2. Because you want to be successful and prove to the nurse executive and yourself that you can manage this team, where do you begin? Outline the first four steps. Do any other critical issues need to be addressed early on as the new team leader?
3. All teams progress through certain stages as they mature. What are those stages, and what are the hallmarks of each stage?
4. In reviewing all the team members, how would the team leader assist each person in turning from a dysfunctional to a

functional member? What are some of the techniques to apply
as stated in the text? Do you have the right members on the
team? In what stage of the group process is the group currently
engaged?

5. The team leader is responsible for ensuring that the goals of
the team are accomplished. How can one run the most effective meeting? Identify at least six key factors in evaluating a
team's progress toward meeting their goals and objectives.

Case Analysis

1. As the newly assigned team leader, do you feel challenged or
overwhelmed?

   Everyone feels overwhelmed at first in a new setting,
especially with a team that has not been 100% successful.
Hopefully, the feelings of being overwhelmed will not
immobilize the new team leader and, instead, will offer much
in the way of a challenge: How can he or she best motivate
the team members to carry out the vision that has been
determined for the team?

2. Because you want to be successful and prove to the nurse
executive and yourself that you can manage this team, where
do you begin? Outline the first four steps. Do any other critical
issues need to be addressed early on as the new team leader?

   Before anything else, take a deep breathe and repeat to
yourself, "I can do this!" Understand that change is not made
overnight, that not everyone wants to be an equal team
member, and that not everyone has the same goals for even
being on the team.

   The first place to start is to make sure the meeting has a
clear agenda and reason. Many committees and teams met
simply because they always have and really do have no
specific agenda other than "We've always done it this way!" A
fair amount can be accomplished within the group setting, and
the responsibility of the team leader is to ensure that the team
has a clear purpose and goal to attain. Otherwise, why should
there be a meeting, and what should be accomplished?

   The second issue is to choose the team members wisely.
Some members are assigned for political reasons or because
of their status or power from within the organization. Others
need to be there because of what they can bring to the team.

Should there be members from one specialty area, is there a need for interdisciplinary members, and is there a need for specialty and professional representation?

Ensure that a clearly identified method of communication is in place. Who will take minutes at the meetings? How quickly will they be completed and distributed? How will they be distributed? How will decisions that require a fast answer be made? If you choose e-mail as the communication method, does everyone read them? Are meetings set in advance to allow members to adjust their schedules ahead of time?

As the team leader, you need to ensure that all members are actively participating in achieving the team's goals and objectives. Some members may be more active than others or have a task that may hold more responsibility; however, all need to feel like they are contributing equally.

Finally, but most importantly, the team leader needs to keep the team on track and focused with an action plan that is understood by all members as well as any outside administrators, staff, or other communities of interest. Ongoing assessment and evaluation are continuous throughout the process so that a team does not pursue an unobtainable objective that was doomed to failure from the beginning of the project.

3. All teams progress through certain stages as they mature. What are those stages, and what are the hallmarks of each stage?

The first phase is the forming phase, during which expectations, boundaries, and interactions are the primary issues to discuss with the new group members. No one really knows where the team is going. People may not know one another, and some may be unsure what they are able to contribute to the team's overall success.

After the introductions are made and the team members begin to feel more comfortable verbalizing, the storming phase begins. During this phase, conflict may occur as freer thoughts and ideas are shared. Expectations of others may become more critical as well during this phase of confrontation.

Equilibrium occurs again during the norming phase, in which team members have worked through the majority of the conflict and now want to work on successfully attaining their goals. This norming phase leads to the reason why most people join a team: a sense of camaraderie and accomplishment as the group makes great strides in progress.

When the project is over and the goal has been accomplished, the final stage of adjourning begins. Members evaluate their progress toward meeting the expected goals and objectives during this stage. Closure needs to occur in this phase as well.

4. In reviewing all the team members, how would the team leader assist each person in turning from a dysfunctional to a functional member? What are some of the techniques to apply as stated in the text? Do you have the right members on the team? In what stage of the group process is the group currently engaged?

One of the most critical jobs for the team leader is to keep the team members on track and on task. Some members may not be conscious of the role that they are playing; others are very aware of their actions. At this point, it is too early to tell whether all the members are appropriate for the team, because the first meeting attended by the newly assigned team leader has turned out to be fairly nonproductive, with the team apparently stuck between the forming and storming phases of the group process.

Jamie is a pleaser who wants to be liked, regardless of what his real opinions are. You need to make sure he doesn't volunteer for too much, become overloaded, and eventually, burn out and lose enthusiasm.

Angela is a detailer who needs to have all the information in front of her before she will even attempt to make a decision. Allow her to participate in keeping the team on track. She can provide the meeting's objective for the session and review the past minutes and past decisions. A downfall to detailers is that they sometimes need to think about the ideas on the table before they offer an opinion, so they may slow down group decisions. It can be helpful, however, to have them research, ahead of time, the different options that will be presented.

Samantha may not even be interested in attending the meeting, and she acts out in a passive manner. As the team leader, you need to ask her privately if she does, in fact, want to participate on the team. If she does, then ask her not to bring her charting so that she can devote her full attention to the meeting at hand, because you value her input. When dealing with a passive personality, it is best to ask direct rather than open-ended questions.

Annabelle is quiet and soft-spoken, yet she wants to keep the group focused and going in the right direction. As the team leader, you need to help her to be heard, both by involving her and by making sure that others listen to her comments.

Finally, Beth is probably the most difficult personality for most team leaders to work with: the criticizer. This person wants to make themselves look good—often at the expense of others. Do not argue with her, especially in front of the group, because it will only add fuel to fire! It is sometimes best to give a criticizer a project to which they can directly contribute; this way, they have the control that they need. As the team leader, you should ask Beth for her opinions and reflect back what she says. More times than not, the criticizer is correct in what they say, but how they say it makes others not want to actively listen.

5. The team leader is responsible for ensuring that the goals of the team are accomplished. How can one run the most effective meeting? Identify at least six key factors in evaluating the team's progress toward meeting their goals and objectives.

One of the most important things to keep in mind as the team leader is to be *organized*. Do you have the meetings arranged ahead of time? Do you have the room reserved? Are the minutes of the previous meeting distributed for comments before the next meeting? Does the meeting begin and end on time? Team members are more apt to respond positively when they feel the group meeting has an understood purpose and a clear vision regarding the goals and objectives.

The team leader needs to keep a close watch on the dynamics of the group and, as much as possible, minimize the dysfunctional behaviors and conversations to encourage positive decision-making. In doing so, the leader also ensures that all members are contributing in some fashion. Contributions are not always equal, of course, but all members should participate. Likewise, especially in brainstorming sessions, mutual support rather than criticism of new ideas should be encouraged.

Is the meeting productive? Does the group see actual progress toward meeting their goals and objectives? Although there may be impediments to progress at several steps along the way, some gain should be measurable.

What type of leader are you? Do you provide energy and enthusiasm for the group? Were you selected against your will? Do you provide a vision for where the team needs to go? People will respond positively when they see your passion for improvement, whether it be regarding a situation (e.g., decreasing patient falls) or a procedure (e.g., hanging blood) or even improving communications between different shifts. The team leader is responsible for making sure that the group knows where they are going, in terms of goals and objectives, and what they still need to accomplish.

Case Scenario 10-2

You are the charge nurse on the weekend, and you have noticed an increase in patient complaints about the food service during the last 3 months. Of particular concern are the trays that are not even opened for the patients or the trays that are left out of reach. For example, you went into Mr. Wen's room, and his tray was placed unopened on the windowsill. Mr. Wen, who does not speak English, looked at you and pointed to the tray when you walked into the room. It was already 1:30 PM. The trays were supposed to be picked up by 1:00 PM, but no one from dietary showed up until after 2:15 PM. One of the nursing assistants began stacking the dirty trays at the nurses' station, eliciting complaints from the two physicians who needed to use the dictation equipment.

When you approach your nurse manager, he says that this would be a great opportunity for you to begin using more of your leadership abilities to solve this problem.

One of the first things you remember from your leadership and management class is to ask others for their input to solicit change. Doing a quick survey of the staff nurses on the weekends, you find out the following information:

1. The trays are not delivered at any specific time. Instead, they arrive for each meal with a great deal of time variability.
2. The dietary staff appears to be short-staffed.
3. The dietary staff is often uncomfortable entering a patient's room, much less engaging a patient or their family in conversation.
4. Trays are left unopened or not within reach of a patient.
5. Trays often are not picked up in a timely manner or are left on the unit for the next mealtime.
6. Nursing assistants do not always remove the trays when they have the opportunity. At other times, they stack them wherever they find room, such as clean and dirty utility rooms or the

nurses' station. Once, you even found trays in a vacant patient room.

Case Considerations

1. Were you able to solicit information from all the necessary people?
2. Now that you have this information, what are the next steps in solving this issue?
3. What are some practical short-term solutions? What is the longer-term, team development plan?
4. What are some solutions that may take additional training and more time to change?

Case Analysis

When your manager asked you to solve this problem, you began by asking your fellow nurses about the situation, which was a great beginning. Now, you need to include others who can directly effect the change and devise both short- and long-term solutions.

■ KEY POINTS

1. To make an informed decision, you need to have all the necessary information from all the right people. You began with the nurses, but who else do you need to include in this change to see the whole picture? Who do you not need to include? Are different shifts and days of the week important to consider?
2. Now that you have information from a variety of people, you need to think about the next steps. Is this a problem that you can solve by yourself, or do you need others to assist? What are the most important issues to resolve? What are some of the issues that really don't require that an immediate change occur? How will you prioritize?
3. What are some of the issues for which you cannot wait to get everyone's buy-in and approval? What are some of the issues that can be addressed by a flyer, and what are some of the issues that may need to wait until a staff meeting? What are the specific patient issues that need to be changed immediately? Do any issues require help from other departments?
4. Some issues in this case will take retraining, because they may be related to a knowledge deficit or an accumulation of bad

habits. What are these issues? Who needs the training, and how will you make sure that it is provided? When your manager asks how long some of these retraining sessions will take, what is your response? How would you ensure that change has occurred?

Case Scenario 10-3

Amanda, one of the registered nurses (RNs) on the assisted living unit where you work, has become more difficult to work with lately. Amanda is your preceptor; however, it is hard to get her to help you with much. At times, she can be curt and critical; at other times, she can be helpful. Amanda directs you to work with the two nursing assistants on your team or with the licensed practical nurse (LPN); she tells you that was how she learned as a new employee. Although you value the roles and knowledge of assistants and the LPN, you feel that you really need assistance in the professional responsibilities, such as delegating, passing medications, taking verbal orders, and speaking with physicians.

The two nursing assistants and the LPN are having some issues with Amanda as well. She does not readily share treatment plans, so many times the goals and objectives for the client are unknown. The assistants and the LPN tell you that they would like to become more of a team rather than being on their own as much as they are, and they would also like more guidance. Because you are the newest member, they ask you to speak to Amanda on their behalf.

Case Considerations

1. What are the issues at hand?
2. Would you speak with Amanda? Why, or why not? Is this an important issue? If you choose to speak with Amanda, what will your game plan be?
3. What would Amanda's perception most likely be regarding this situation?
4. How would you include the other team members in the discussion?
5. Devise a team development plan.

Case Analysis

Communication issues can be especially hard to deal with, especially with a variety of team members involved.

■ *KEY POINTS*

1. What are they key issues for you to discuss? It is important that you have a clear idea about the issues at hand, not just a perception that you are being ignored. Also, clearly differentiate between your issues and the team's issues. Are they the same? Are they different? How have they coped in the past with these issues? How has Amanda responded in the past to requests, or have no requests been made?
2. What are the potential repercussions if you speak with Amanda about your concerns? What are the repercussions if you do not speak with Amanda? What are the risks either way?
3. The others want you to speak with Amanda on their behalf, but what are the risks in doing so at this point? What are the risks if you do not? If you choose to speak on their behalf, which issues will you include, and why?
4. Before you do anything, make sure that you have all your facts straight. How would you accomplish this task? Would you include only your issues or those of the other team members as well? What are your desired outcomes? How will you know if you are successful? How would you begin the conversation? Who else would be there? Where would the conversation be?

Suggested Readings

Bennis, W. (1989). *Why leaders can't lead.* San Francisco: Jossey-Bass.
Brown, B. (1998). 10 Trends for the new year: Nurse managers predict the skills and mind-set you'll need to prosper in 1999. *Nursing Management, 29* (2), 33–36.
Burns, J. M. (1978). *Leadership.* New York: Harper & Row.
Davis, B. L., Hellervik, L. W., Sheard, J. L., Skube, C. J., & Gebelein, S. H. (1996). *Manager's Handbook.* Minneapolis: Personnel Decisions International.
Harwood, A. (1997). Spot the saboteurs. *Nursing Times, 93* (25), 72–75.
Hunsaker, P. L., & Alessandra, A. J. (1980). *The art of managing people.* Englewood Cliffs, NJ: Prentice Hall.
Katzenbach, J. R., & Smith, D. K. (1993). *The wisdom of teams: Creating the high-performance organization.* New York: Harper Business.
Lacoursier, R. B. (1980). *The life cycle of groups: Group development stage theory.* New York: Human Sciences Press.
Leppa, C. J. (1996). Nurse relationships and work group disruptions. *Journal of Nursing Administration, 26* (10), 23–27.
Marquis, B. L., & Huston, C. J. (2000). *Leadership roles and management functions in nursing.* Philadelphia: J. B. Lippincott.

McGregor, D. (1960). *The human side of enterprise.* New York: McGraw-Hill.

Prager, H. (1999). Cooking up effective team building. *Training & Development, 53* (12), 14.

Senge, P. M. (1990). *The fifth discipline.* New York: Doubleday Books.

Tuckman, B. W., & Jensen, M. A. (1977). Stages of small group development revisited. *Group and Organizational Studies, 2* (4), 419.

Whittier, S. (1999). Manager's corner: Effective team building: More important than ever. *Home Care Nurse News, 6* (3), 1–3.

Wilson, R. D., Mateo, M. A., & Brumm, S. K. (1999). Revitalizing a departmental committee. *Journal of Nursing Administration, 29* (3), 45–48.

Chapter 11

Budget Concepts for Patient Care

Essential Concepts in Budgeting for Patient Care

Like any service, successful health care delivery depends on resources of money, people, supplies, and equipment. To ensure that staff have these resources to manage patient care, the nurse manager is accountable for planning and implementing a budget along with other financial resources within an organization. Given all the variables, maintaining a budget, once approved, is often a challenge. A budget needs to be reviewed on at least a monthly basis, with the manager and others examining its variability based on actual events, revenue, and expenses. Staffing issues are generally reviewed for variance on a daily basis.

The budget is comprised of two primary areas, the operational budget and the capital budget. The operational budget is the one over which a nurse manager has the most control, because it contains labor, supplies, and equipment. The operational budget also includes revenue; however, most managers do not have control over or input into this section of the budget. The capital budget is comprised of items such as new or replacement equipment that are not considered to be disposable. Some organizations include new construction within the capital budget; others have a separate budget and process for new construction.

Budget Types

- Operational budgets are the day-to-day accounting of what monies are brought in by the organization (revenues) and what monies are needed to provide services (costs).
- Revenues generate billable services and the costs associated with running the business of health care, including labor, equipment, testing, supplies, and indirect costs (e.g., building maintenance).
- Revenues are based on the type of procedure that a patient has and how many days (or even hours) that he or she needs to use the facility, staff, and equipment.
- When devising an operational budget, staffing, patient days, costs of doing business, and any new projects are calculated into the total amount.
- Some facilities separate the labor portion of the operational budget and devise a separate personnel budget. Historically, nursing personnel have been the largest component of hospital labor budgets.
- A capital budget is specifically for those major, nondisposable purchases that an organization makes during its fiscal year. To classify a piece of new or replacement equipment as capital, it must cost more than a certain amount of money and have a projected expected life span.
- When an immense renovation or building project occurs, a separate construction budget may be devised to contain all the costs needed to complete the project.

Budget Preparation Process

- The first step in any budgeting process is to understand thoroughly the fundamentals that influence generally the organization and, more specifically, the unit for which the budget is being developed.
- The information needed during the budget preparation period includes the scope of service, goals, demographic information, patient days, staffing patterns and skill mix, and provider profiles. The services offered are reviewed, and trends are examined to ensure at least maintenance, if not growth, in patient admissions to the unit.
- Often, a competitive analysis is completed before the budgeting process begins to assess how competing health care organizations are performing compared to your facility. A review of provider

practices, patient days, strengths and weaknesses, and new services
is completed to assist the manager in making informed decisions
before recommending a new product line or the hiring of new staff.
- Regulatory bodies, such as the Centers for Medicare and Medicaid
Services (www.cms.hhs.gov), the U.S. Food and Drug Administration (www.fda.gov), and the Joint Commission on the Accreditation
of Healthcare Agencies (http://www.jcaho.org), play a role in
reimbursement rates that affect the financial performance of an
organization.
- The organization's goals and objectives, often implemented through
a strategic plan, guide the development of a unit's budget.

Cost Centers

- A cost center is the smallest functional unit for which costs and
accountability can be attributed.

Budget Development

- In developing a budget, it is important to identify the amount of
projected revenue compared to the current year. Reimbursement
rates from third-party payers, such as insurance companies, affect
the amount of expected revenue and depend on services provided,
patient days, and any discounts to the organization.
- Reimbursement rates and percentages also vary by provider and
type of patient using the facilities, and they often change yearly
(Figure 11-1). These payers determine what costs are allowable
for each procedure or service, and they reimburse the hospital
or provider accordingly. The diagnostic related group (DRG)
classification system is used to classify patients by diagnosis,
with each diagnosis predesignated a certain allowable charge for
inpatient days.
- Capitation is the fixed, preset payment for a certain service to one
person for a specific time.
- Expenses are the costs that are necessary to provide the services of
the health care setting. Supply inventories are analyzed for historical, current, and projected use.
- Direct expenses are directly associated with the costs of taking care
of patients, including supplies, drugs, and medical gases. Indirect
costs are more difficult to calculate, such as utilities, building maintenance, housekeeping, and even nursing care.
- Fixed costs are expenses that do not change according to patient
volume or productivity levels. Variable costs are affected by patient

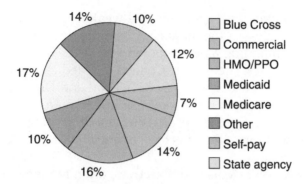

The reimbursement rates vary depending on
the payer. For example, Medicare may reimburse
40% of charges, Medicaid's rate may be 30%,
and managed care may be 60%. Factoring in
reimbursement rates leads to profit and loss
calculations for an organization.

Figure 11-1   Inpatient Payer Mix.

volume and productivity levels. For example, one can always expect
more laundry if a unit is full versus half-full.
- Labor costs are often significant in health care, with professional
  staff often being the most costly. With today's environment of
  recruitment and retention, especially of registered nurses (RNs) and
  other allied health professionals, a manager must look critically at
  projected costs, at actual salary costs, and at the costs of marketing
  and recruiting new staff.
- Staffing issues in an acute care setting are often complex. Productive
  time includes the time during which a staff member is actually
  providing direct care. Unproductive time is also considered when
  devising a budget, and it includes nonpatient care time, such as
  vacation, education, personal, and holiday time.

Budget Approval and Monitoring

- Often, a budget is in the development stage for 3 to 6 months. Once
  the development stage has been completed, the budget moves on
  to the approval phase. During the approval phase, the appropriate
  administrator confers with necessary finance individuals who
  review the entire organization's budgets.
- Once approved and distributed, the budget is usually monitored for
  variances on a monthly basis. A variance can be either positive or

negative, but both types generally need an explanation. The department manager is responsible for maintaining the budget and controlling the costs to the best of his or her ability. This is a critical area of responsibility for the nurse manager, because controlling expenses, particularly in the area of staffing, have a direct impact on the bottom-line revenues of the hospital. In fact, many hospitals employ a full-time budget analyst specifically for the Nursing Department to ensure that these expenses are carefully monitored and evaluated.

Miscellaneous Budgeting Concepts

- The case mix consists of the types and varieties of patients who are admitted into an inpatient setting. Examples of a case mix include patient diagnoses by DRGs or insurance payment types.
- Just as the case mix describes the types of patients who are found within an institution, the staffing mix describes the varieties of staff who are employed. For example, a staffing mix for a medical-surgical unit may be 40% RNs, 40% licensed practical nurses (LPNs), and 20% unlicensed assistive personnel (UAPs).
- An employee is characterized as being either full-time or part-time, with their calculated time compared to a full-time equivalent (FTE). Generally, someone who works 40 hours a week for 52 weeks a year and, thus, works 2,080 hours a year and is considered to hold one FTE position.
- The nursing care hours provided in one 24-hour period per patient are calculated in a general formula known as hours per patient day (HPPD). This figure is derived by dividing the total numbers of hours worked by the RN by the number of patients in a specific unit.

CASE SCENARIOS

Guided Case Scenario 11-1

You have been asked to develop a new medical-surgical unit, because of an expansion in patient care services, in a pre-existing area of your hospital. Currently, you manage one 20-bed medical-surgical unit, with a focus on chronic medical patients. You meet with your Chief Nursing Officer (CNO), who asks you to develop a tentative operational budget. The unit will be 30 beds, with an emphasis on surgical rather than medical patients.

Here are some facts to work with: Because the new unit will be housed in a designated, pre-existing area of the hospital, which 30 years ago held patients, one does not have to worry about significant construction costs and schedules. Some changes, however, may be needed to accommodate surgical patients and to update the rooms.

Other areas of the hospital, with the exception of pediatrics, are also experiencing full census, so there may be a limited amount of staff available to bring into the new unit from the existing staff. Extensive recruitment and retention programs are already in place at the hospital in an effort to fill and maintain current positions.

It is expected that you will be the nurse manager of this unit as well as the other medical-surgical unit.

Case Considerations

1. Where does one begin? How does one break down this project into manageable parts?
2. Whom should assist you in this process?
3. Describe the components of the budget that need to be developed and their impact on the new unit.
4. Identify the personnel component of the budget. What should be considered when developing this section of the operational budget?
5. Supplies and equipment are another component of the operational budget. What considerations do you have for this area, and why?
6. Because the new unit is to be housed in a pre-existing area of the hospital, what are your concerns, especially regarding capital requests?

Case Analysis

1. Where does one begin? How does one break down this project into manageable parts?

The key to success in a new project such as this is to look at the entire project as a whole and then begin to separate it into categories. At this point, it may be prudent to secure the assistance of someone who can work with you and, perhaps, even to delegate some areas to others who are qualified to assist.

The different components to developing a new unit include: (1) the physical space and its adequacy for taking patients; (2) equipment and supply needs and availability; (3) staffing and scheduling, including the correct staff mix and ratios; (4) staff training; (5) admission, discharge, and transfer criteria for the new patient population; and (6) development of an operational and capital budget to accomplish the above tasks.

Once the tasks have been divided, you can begin by gathering the information and data that are needed to understand fully the needs of each area. For example, building and maintenance personnel will need to be involved with checking out the allocated physical space: Is it adequate? Does it have the appropriate gas lines? Is there a nurse call system? Is there any need for telemetry? Is there a central nursing station, or does it have modular stations? Does the unit meet all the federal and state regulations necessary for patient occupancy? Is there room for clean and dirty utility rooms, a nursing station, a medication preparation and storage area, and break room? All these questions can be answered by involving the correct personnel early in the process rather than waiting until a problem arises. In a large project such as this, it is imperative to spend adequate time at the beginning by planning rather than simply jumping in and starting a little bit of everything.

2. Whom should assist you in this process?

After identifying the different components needed to successfully accomplish this project, it would be helpful to connect with someone having specific knowledge about that area. As in the above example, it will be necessary to involve the physical plant supervisor early in the process, especially if the area has construction needs. Who else would be helpful? The staffing office, the Education Department, central supply, the pharmacy—everyone who has potential to affect patient care should be involved.

3. Describe the components of the budget that need to be developed and their impact on the new unit.

At the very beginning, you need to be concerned with several key areas of the operational budget. One component is the supply and equipment budget, because you are creating a new unit without any supplies or equipment. Another area is the staffing component of the budget, because you must ensure that you have adequate coverage and the proper skill mix to deliver quality care to the patients. Is there any money for education of the staff, particularly if you may be taking some pre-existing staff who wish to transfer but who do not possess the appropriate skills?

4. Identify the personnel component of the budget. What should be considered when developing this section of the operational budget?

   One consideration that almost all budgets begin with is adequate coverage. Adequate coverage is defined differently in every hospital, but the overall goal is to ensure that quality care can be delivered with the available resources. What type of nursing model will this floor follow? Team nursing? Modular nursing? Primary nursing? What is the staffing mix or percentage of RNs to LPNs? Will there be UAPs, and if so, how many? Will there be a secretary on the unit during every shift, including weekends?

   Additionally, when developing a personnel section, strong consideration needs to be given to the nursing workload, or the HPPD. In other words, how much time is the nurse expected to be at the bedside delivering care, and what acuity level is expected of the patients? Generally, on a medical-surgical unit, it is common to have between 4 and 6 hours of nursing care per patient per day. All of these items factor into how much staff, and what level of staffing, will be needed in a personnel budget.

5. Supplies and equipment are another component of the operational budget. What considerations do you have for this area, and why?

   Because this unit is being developed from the beginning, one will need to either purchase new supplies or equipment or look for these items in other areas of the hospital where they can be spared. Either way, one needs to come up with a working list. Generally, supplies are disposable items, such as tape, tubing, and dressing materials. Equipment includes items that can be reused on different patients. Intravenous and pharmacy supplies are needed. Keep in mind, however, that assistance from the pharmacy or central supply will be needed, and it is much easier to do so at the beginning of the project.

6. Because the new unit is to be housed in a pre-existing area of the hospital, what are your concerns, especially when regarding capital requests?

As discussed above, one will need to get building and maintenance involved with checking out the "new" space, because they must ensure that it meets all the federal and state regulations necessary for patient occupancy. After the necessary space has been defined, including firewalls and access to the unit in case of emergency, they can begin working on the more aesthetic areas, such as the nursing station and break room, to enhance work on the unit. It is always a good idea to have nursing involved rather early in these types of decisions, especially to look at the length of the hallways and the locations of patient rooms in conjunction with the nursing station and other necessary supply areas.

Case Scenario 11-2

Your assistant nurse manager has indicated that he would like to learn more about the budgeting process for the bone marrow transplant unit that you manage. As his manager, you would like to make the presentation as logical as possible while making sure that certain necessary components are not missed. Because it is currently the time of the year when the next year's budgets are being developed, you plan to include him in the preparation process as much as can be facilitated.

Case Considerations

1. Discuss the key areas for one to consider when preparing a budget.
2. What documents can be shown to the assistant nurse manager that illustrates the budget and the budgeting process?
3. Identify a tentative timeline for the budgeting process.
4. The assistant nurse manager can certainly contribute to the budgeting process. Describe those areas that would be appropriate for his assistance and input.

Case Analysis

The budgeting process should be understood as a process to which everyone, including staff and other managers on the unit, can contribute. When more people are involved with understanding budget component as well as in developing the budget, the more likelihood there will be of maintaining a healthy bottom line.

▣ *KEY POINTS*

1. Begin by assessing the assistant nurse manager's understanding of the budgeting process.
2. Gather all the appropriate documents that illustrate the different components of the budgeting process, including the capital budget.
3. Ask for the assistant nurse manager's input. Does he see areas that can be pared back a little or that need to have additional funding to increase quality services?
4. Can any parts of the presentation be brought to the staff nurses?
5. Who else could be involved with the budgeting process on the unit, and why?
6. How can the assistant nurse manager be involved with the budgeting process throughout the year, not just at budget preparation time? What key functions can he carry out as part of his job responsibilities?

Case Scenario 11-3

As nurse manager of the outpatient clinic, you have just completed reviewing the budget, which is 3 months into the new fiscal year. You notice a positive variance for medical supplies on your unit—a 45% variance, in fact. The CNO asks you for an in-depth variance report, requesting specifics on why the budget is 45% over in these areas this past quarter.

Case Considerations

1. Describe the variance process and its impact on the yearly budgeting process.
2. What are some possible causes for a 45% variance in the medical supply budget?
3. Is 45% a "normal" variance 3 months into a budget year?
4. Who else could you get involved with the report to the CNO?
5. Identify several steps that can be taken to curtail this overage.

Case Analysis

One of the most important functions of a manager, other than developing a budget for the unit, is to maintain the budget. It is simply not enough to develop a budget and then wait until the end of the fiscal year to see how close one came to the projections.

■ *KEY POINTS*

1. When looking at a budget, it is necessary to review both the year-to-date information, as well as the overall total budget, on a monthly basis. Staffing variances usually are reviewed daily.
2. It is important to review variances as soon as they arise, so that memory does not fade!
3. Sometimes, it takes great detective work to find out where the variance occurred. Do not be discouraged if the answer is hidden among other costs.

Suggested Readings

Barratt, C., & Schultz, M. (1997). Staffing in the operating room: Time and space factors. *Journal of Nursing Administration, 27,* 27–31.

Bryant, J. (2003). A message for budget planners. *Australian Nursing Journal, 10* (8), 3.

Carter, M (2000). Use of a nursing labor productivity measurement tool. *Economic$, 18* (4), 237–242.

Carter, M. (2002). Rural nurse manager's use of a labor computer decision support system. *Nursing Economic$, 20* (5), 237–243.

Daft., R. L., & Marcic, D. (2001). *Understanding management* (3rd ed.). Philadelphia: Harcourt College.

Felteau, A. L. (1992). Budget variance analysis and justification. *Nursing Management, 3* (2): 40–41.

Finkler, S. A. (2001). *Budgeting concepts for nurse managers* (3rd ed.). Philadelphia: W. B. Saunders.

Finkler, D. A., & Kovner, C. T. (2000). *Financial management for nurse managers and executives* (2nd ed.). Philadelphia: W. B. Saunders.

Griggith, J. (1999). *The well-managed health care organization.* Chicago: Health Administration Press.

Henderson, E. (2003). Budgeting: Part One. *Nursing Management, 10* (1), 33–37.

Henderson, E. (2003). Budgeting: Part Two. *Nursing Management, 10* (2), 32–36.

Kirkby, M. B. (2002). Number crunching with variable budgets. *Nursing Management, 34* (3), 28–33.

Kongstvedt, P. (2001). *Essentials in managed care* (4th ed.). Gaithersburg, MD: Aspen Publishers.

Kongstvedt, P. (2002). *Managed care: What it is and how it works.* Gaithersburg, MD: Aspen Publishers.

Lang, N. M. (1999). Discipline approaches to evidence-based practice: A view from nursing. *Joint Commission Journal on Quality Improvement, 25* (10), 539–544.

Marquis, B. L., & Huston, C. J. (2000). *Leadership roles and management functions* (3rd ed.). Philadelphia: J. B. Lippincott.

Meyer, M. A. (1999). An OR staffing guideline: Preparing the OR staff budget. *Surgical Services Management, 5* (8), 42–44.

Moore, K., Lynn, M., McMillen, B., & Evans, S. (1999). Implementation of the ANA report card. *Journal of Nursing Administration, 29* (6), 48–54.

Paprocki, J. S. (2000). Budgeting principles for nurse managers. *DNA Reporter, 25* (1), 18–23.

Reilly, P. (2003). Moving up. Top nurses take on more executive duties as they work their way up. *Modern Healthcare, 33* (13), 12–13.

Shortell, S., & Kaluzny, A. (2000). *Health care management: Organization design and behavior* (4th ed.). Clifton Park, NY: Delmar Learning.

Wolper, L. (1999). *Health care administration planning, implementing and managing organized delivery systems* (3rd ed.). Gaithersburg, MD: Aspen Publishers.

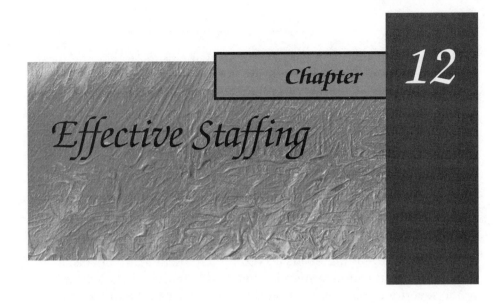

Essential Concepts in Effective Staffing

Staffing is often one of the more challenging functions for a nurse manager. A staffing schedule often depends on the availability and flexibility of qualified staff as well as on the acuity levels of the patients. It is imperative that the manager keep in mind, when developing a staffing pattern, patient safety and delivery of quality patient care. Many tools are available to assist the nurse in providing safe and effective care, including patient classification systems, benchmarking data, and regulatory requirements.

In developing a staffing pattern, the nurse manager requires certain pieces of information before he or she can effectively plan. Necessary information includes data on the unit itself, such as how many beds are available for occupancy, the occupancy rate, the general layout, and so on. Skill mix is determined early in the process, as are the nursing hours per patient day (NHPPD) that will be used in patient care delivery. Staff experience also needs to be kept in mind when developing a schedule, especially if new graduates, who need extra mentoring and guidance, are to be included. In meeting the needs of both the staff and the patient, several models of nursing care can be used, including total patient care, team nursing, primary nursing, patient-focused care, differentiated practice, functional nursing, and the case method of patient care.

Core Concepts of Effective Staffing

- The core concepts of full-time equivalents (FTEs), productive and nonproductive hours, direct and indirect care, and NHPPD are all necessary terms in understanding how to develop, assess, and evaluate a staffing pattern.

Patient Classification Systems

- To determine staffing needs according to patient acuity levels, a patient classification system is often used. Acuity levels determine the severity of patient needs and the workload of the nurse in caring for those patients.
- When a manager uses a patient classification system to plan for staffing needs, each patient is categorized according to the nursing care hours that will be needed during a 24-hour period. These nursing care hours include bathing, ambulation, supervision, assessment, treatments, and medication administration.
- Data generated from a patient classification system assists the manager in monitoring nurse-staffing levels, patient acuities, and variances in staff utilization.

Developing a Staffing Pattern

- Developing a staffing pattern for a unit requires several key pieces of information, such as regulatory requirements, skill mix, staff support, and historical information.
- Several states have specific staffing requirements, such as how many registered nurses (RNs) must be present on a shift.
- Skill mix is the delineation of skill levels on a nursing unit, which may include RNs, licensed practical nurses (LPNs), aides, and other support personnel. Skill mix also depends on the care setting: A skilled nursing facility will use a lower ratio of RNs to patients than a critical care unit will use.
- Staff support is important to review when considering how many other "duties" other than direct patient care, such as obtaining medications, taking patients to radiology, and providing secretarial support, the professional staff will need to fulfill.
- When devising a staffing pattern, the best place to start is often with historical information. What were the types of patients? What were

Skill	Day	Evening	Night	Total
Direct				
ANM				
RN	4	3.5	3	10.5
LPN				
Tech				
UAP	2	1.5	1	4.5
Subtotal				

10.5 staff × 8-hour shifts   =   120 hours
4.5 staff × 8-hour shifts   =   36 hours

Staff hours available per day =   156 hours

156 hours ÷ 22 patients per day = 7.09 hours of NHPPD

156 hours ÷   8-hour shifts   = 19.5 FTEs to fill the staffing pattern

Figure 12-1   Staffing Plan for a 24-Bed Medical Unit.

the staffing patterns? Did the staffing patterns meet the needs of the patients and the staff?

- An example of a staffing plan is shown in Figure 12-1.

Evaluating Staffing Effectiveness

- When evaluating staffing effectiveness, patient and nursing outcomes should be the first priorities. Did the patients receive the care that was ordered in a timely, efficient, and quality manner? Did the nurses who provided the care feel that they gave competent, quality care?
- Turnover rates are also reviewed as part of evaluating staffing effectiveness. Turnover is caused by many factors, including staff satisfaction levels and transfers either to another unit or out of the institution entirely.

Models of Care Delivery

- In the case method, the nurse cares for a patient's entire needs in a holistic manner. The case method is also known as total patient care, in which an RN may be assigned only a few patients but is responsible for all assessments, treatments, medication administrations, and other necessary concerns. Many intensive care units use the total patient care model and may have assistants in the form of aides or LPNs.

- Functional nursing divides tasks or assigns specific duties according to the skill level of the provider. For example, an evening shift may have a medication nurse, treatment nurse, and charge nurse, plus an aide who provides all personal care.
- Team nursing has been the most popular model in recent years, with many known hybrids. A team is assigned a group of patients, with one of the team RNs acting as the team leader, who is responsible for the coordination of all the care of these patients. Care is usually assigned according to the skill level of the provider, with teams often consisting of LPNs and aides and, possibly, an RN. Both team nursing and functional nursing are the least expensive types of care delivery models being used in health care facilities, because the staffing patterns have RNs, LPNs, and unlicensed assistive personnel (UAPs). The quality with these models, however, must be closely supervised, because fewer RNs are providing direct patient care.
- Primary nursing is much like total patient care but has additional components. In primary nursing, each patient is assigned to an RN on his or her admission, and this nurse stays with the patient throughout the hospitalization, giving the primary nurse total accountability, authority, and responsibility for the nursing care provided. This type of care delivery model, along with case management, is one of the most expensive, because many RNs are needed to be the primary care givers. These models, however, also have the highest levels of both RN satisfaction and quality outcomes.
- In patient-focused care, the care is provided based on the needs of the patient, with many services coming to the patient rather than the patient going to the services. For example, in a patient-focused environment, basic physical therapy services may be offered on each patient floor, eliminating the need for transporting the patient off the floor for services. Often, other disciplines are involved in direct patient care activities that may not have been as closely involved in the past; for example, housekeeping may be cross-trained to deliver patient trays.
- With differentiated practice, the RN performs skills and functions according to identified criteria, most commonly education, practice, and competency. Differentiated practice often rewards nurses who achieve certain educational degrees (e.g., the BSN) with additional incentives and recognition.

Case Management

- A primary role of the case manager is to coordinate the care of a patient throughout his or her hospitalization. The case manager establishes daily goals for the patient to meet and evaluates of whether the patient has achieved these goals.
- A tool that many case managers use to evaluate whether a patient has met his or her daily goals is the clinical pathway, in which patient outcomes are identified. Many clinical pathways are inter-disciplinary in nature, allowing not only nursing but also social work, dietary, physical therapy, and other disciplines to coordinate the care of a patient. Patient progress is measured and evaluated daily.

CASE SCENARIOS

Guided Case Scenario 12-1

As the nurse manager of a 20-bed medical-surgical unit, one of your primary responsibilities is to ensure adequate staffing and ap-propriate staff mix on the unit. This year has seen a fair amount of turnover for a variety to reasons, including a new hospital that opened nearby with a substantial hiring bonus. Many new RN graduates were hired because of these vacancies.

It has always been the unit's policy to work out the Thanksgiv-ing/Christmas/New Year's schedule before Halloween. Many of the senior staff worked the Christmas holiday last year and are requesting to work the New Year's holiday this year. The majority of the new staff members only want to work the New Year's holi-day, and they are threatening to leave if they have to work the Christmas holiday. Because this is a busy unit, closing is not an option. The unit needs to be fully staffed during all three holidays.

Case Considerations

1. Because closing the unit and granting everyone the holiday that they desire is clearly not possible, come up with at least three options for the holiday schedule.
2. Are the senior staff who have been with employed on the unit for many years favored, or are the new staff nurses, whom you don't want to lose to another place of employment, favored?

3. Which of the three options that you derived benefits the most people? Which option benefits the fewest? Which option do you believe is the right choice, and why?
4. How would one implement the chosen option?
5. How would one evaluate the chosen option as a success or as a failure?

Case Analysis

1. Because closing the unit and granting everyone the holiday that they desire is clearly not possible, come up with at least three options for the holiday schedule.

   Sometimes, in producing a schedule, some people are never satisfied and others, as long as they receive their requested time, do not seem to mind what is developed. In this particular scenario, a potential crisis looms, with the decision made about the staffing pattern in question having the potential to affect future schedules as well.

   Several different options need to be considered when a scenario such as this arises. Option A is to assign half the staff to work Christmas and the other half to work New Year's by seniority. Option B is to assign half the staff to work Christmas and the other half to work New Year's alphabetically. Option C is to assign half the staff to work Christmas and the other half to work New Year's by drawing names out of a hat. Option D is to assist the staff in doing their own schedule to have half the staff working Christmas and the other half working the New Year's holiday. Option E is to do nothing (this is always an option!). The most important thing to remember is to involve the staff in the decision-making process.

2. Are the senior staff who have been employed on the unit for many years favored, or are the new staff nurses, whom you don't want to lose to another place of employment, favored?

   One of the issues is how to reward those who have been loyal to the hospital and the unit for many years. One does not want to alienate them by favoring the new staff; however, you are quite aware that the hiring bonuses from the other hospital are lucrative and a threat to keeping your current staff.

   Are there some rewards that the hospital can implement for the senior staff? Many facilities have not only recruitment committees but also retention committees to focus on these issues. Should senior staff receive a more favorable schedule? Did they begin on a shift that was not their first choice but later moved off it? Should all new nurses "pay their dues" with rotating schedules or off-shifts, or should they be given what they desire to recruit them? These are tough decisions with potential to affect morale, productivity, and retention of the entire nursing staff, so the prudent nurse manager will be extra cautious when making these particular staffing decisions.

3. Which of the three options that you derived benefits the most people? Which option benefits the fewest? Which option do you believe is the right choice, and why?

    Clearly, Option E is not possible at this point, so it is eliminated. Option A benefits the more senior staff. With Option A, however, the manager needs to be concerned with the experience level that will be available on the undesirable holiday.

    Option B really is the most basic, but it does not take into account the senior staff who may have worked last Christmas. Neither does Option C. Option D is the optimal alternative at this point. Having staff self-schedule may yield some surprises, such as staff actually volunteering for a holiday if they perceive they have control over their schedule.

4. How would one implement the chosen option?

    Option D, or self-scheduling, requires teaching, monitoring, and a final review by the manager. Because self-scheduling involves a learning curve, teaching needs to begin as soon as the decision is made to implement this type of scheduling. Conflicts are decided by the nurse manager and are considered to be final. Changes after the schedule is posted have to be worked out between staff, again with final approval by the manager. Many good articles are available that describe the self-scheduling process and its implementation, and even a committee comprised of staff can be convened to assist the rest of the staff in this new process.

5. How would one evaluate the chosen option as a success or as a failure?

    The best way to assess whether the chosen option is a success or a failure is by how many staff actually show up for their scheduled shift! Other than this, the retention of seasoned as well as new staff is one variable to evaluate, along with the staff's perceptions of whether the chosen alternative is viewed as fair and equitable.

Case Scenario 12-2

Lately, your staff has been asking for a "different" way of delivering patient care, one that is more effective, that is more professional, and that uses the LPNs, RNs, and UAPs more efficiently. Staff are not feeling cohesive, and many gaps in patient care are occurring because of an increasing attitude of "that is not my job."

Currently, the care delivery model being used is a modified functional nursing model, in which someone is assigned medication administration, someone is assigned treatments, someone is assigned AM/PM care, and someone is assigned discussion of patient care with the physician staff.

Case Considerations

1. Now that you have this information about the staff's desire to change their care delivery model, what would be the first step in the process to change models?
2. Who should be involved with this change of models, and why?
3. What models would be a consideration if the staff mix included LPNs, RNs, and UAPs?
4. What models would not be a consideration if the staff mix included LPNs, RNs, and UAPs?
5. Are there any other issues to consider when deciding on a new care delivery model?

Case Analysis

A care delivery model generally assists nursing staff in providing optimal patient care in the most efficient and effective manner using skills from each type of nursing personnel. When evaluating which care delivery model would be appropriate to implement, keep in mind the staff mix, the staff's experience, the acuity level of the patients, the layout of the unit, and the staff's willingness to cooperate as a team.

■ KEY POINTS

1. Functional nursing often disenfranchises staff as it breaks responsibilities into tasks.
2. Team nursing requires a strong RN leader.
3. Modular nursing often is driven by the physical layout of the unit.

4. In patient-focused care, the needed care comes to the patient rather than the patient traveling throughout the hospital. Many personnel are also cross-trained in this model.
5. Primary nursing works particularly well with an all-RN staff who take total responsibility for the 24-hour care of the patient.
6. In the differentiated practice model, care is delegated according to the level of education, competency, and practice ability.

Case Scenario 12-3

A patient classification system is an instrument that measures the acuity and intensity of nursing care, or the nursing workload, required by each patient in a specific unit. The following categories are found at St. Mary's Hospital:

- *Level One Patient:* simple needs, generally ambulatory, simple medications and treatments, vital signs each shift, routine teaching.
- *Level Two Patient:* Level One needs plus catheters; vital signs every 4 hours; needs assistance with ambulation; moderate teaching, including lifestyle changes; medications include evaluations before and after administration.
- *Level Three Patient:* moderate needs that may include the above plus frequent treatments, IVs with medications, invasive procedures, more complex patient teaching that may involve family.
- *Level Four Patient:* Critically ill, requires frequent vital signs, probably not ambulating (or at least not independently), IV therapy with frequent titrations, teaching involves patient and/or family (who may be resistant or severely emotionally reactive).

Case Considerations

1. For each of the four categories, give two examples of what types of patients would be classified within them.
2. What would make a patient increase in acuity for each category?
3. What are some positive points about using a patient classification system to determine staffing needs?
4. What are some negative points about using a patient classification system to determine staffing needs?

Case Analysis

When a hospital uses a patient classification system to assist in determining staffing needs, a predominant focus is predicting the

amount of nursing time that will be needed to take care of a designated group of patients. Many patient classification systems are
used to predict nursing care needs for the next shift, or maybe for
the next 24 hours, with a focus on the patient acuity levels either
rising or decreasing.

■ KEY POINTS

1. Many times, a patient classification system is meant to be a
   predictor of nursing care needs, or nursing workload.
2. A patient may be assessed once a day or once a shift.
3. As a patient's acuity level decreases, he or she needs less nursing care. As the patient's acuity level increases, he or she needs
   more care.
4. Patient classification systems review such patient needs as
   frequency of vital signs, ambulation, treatments and their
   complexity, medications with their complexity and need for
   titration, and patient teaching.
5. Patient classification systems provide important information
   that assists the manager in making staffing decisions on a shift-
   by-shift basis. It can allow the manager to be able to adjust
   staffing patterns based on the acuity levels of the patients in
   the unit.
6. The best patient classification systems are objective, with little
   room for subjectivity and manipulation of the data.
7. The information supplied by the patient classification system
   can also be used to cost-out nursing care services.
8. Certain regulatory bodies, such as the Joint Commission on
   the Accreditation of Health Care Organizations (JCAHO) speak
   directly to the staffing of a health care institution.

Suggested Readings

Aiken, L. H., Sloan, D. M., & Sochalski, J. (1998). Hospital organization and outcomes. *Quality in Healthcare, 7* (4), 222–226.

Blancett, S. S., & Flarey, D. L. (1996). Case studies in nursing case management.
Gaithersburg, MD: Aspen Publishers.

Bower, K. A. (1992). *Case management by nurses.* Washington, D.C.: American
Nurses Publishing.

Daft., R. L., & Marcic, D. (2001). *Understanding management* (3rd ed.). Philadelphia: Harcourt College.

Finkler, S. A. (2001). *Budgeting concepts for nurse managers* (3rd ed.). Philadelphia: W. B. Saunders.

Finkler, D. A., & Kovner, C. T. (2000). *Financial management for nurse managers and executives* (2nd ed.). Philadelphia: W. B. Saunders.

Flarey, D. L., & Blancett, S. S. (1996). *Handbook of nursing case management.* Gaithersburg, MD: Aspen Publishers.

Hickey, J. V., Ouimette, R. M., & Venegoni, S. L. (1996). *Advanced practice nursing.* Philadelphia: J. B. Lippincott.

Griggith, J. (1999). *The well-managed health care organization.* Chicago: Health Administration Press.

Kongstvedt, P. (2001). *Essentials in managed care* (4th ed.). Gaithersburg, MD: Aspen Publishers.

Kongstvedt, P. (2002). *Managed care: What it is and how it works.* Gaithersburg, MD: Aspen Publishers.

Lang, N. M. (1999). Discipline approaches to evidence-based practice: A view from nursing. *Joint Commission Journal on Quality Improvement, 25* (10), 539–544.

Lagoe, R. J. (1998). Basis statistics for clinical pathway evaluation. *Nursing Economic$, 16* (3), 125–131.

Lichtig, L. K., Knaug, R. A., Rison-McCoy, R., & Wozniak, L. M. (2000). *Nurse staffing and patient outcomes in the inpatient hospital setting.* Washington, D.C.: American Nurses Association.

Malloch, K., & Conivaloff, A. (1999). Patient classification systems, part 1. *Journal of Nursing Administration, 29* (7/8), 49–56.

Marquis, B. L., & Huston, C. J. (2000). *Leadership roles and management functions* (3rd ed.). Philadelphia: J. B. Lippincott.

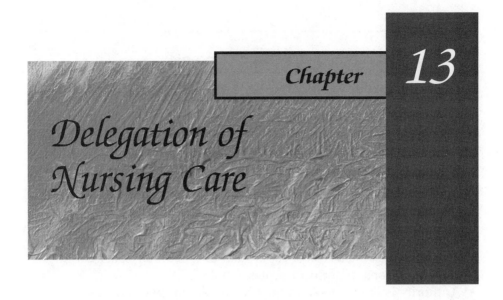

Chapter 13

Delegation of Nursing Care

Essential Concepts in Delegation

Delegation, much like leadership, is the art of accomplishing work through others. Nursing has become so multifaceted that it is difficult for one person to complete every task. Delegation is a skill that is learned, and it is essential in fulfilling the daily responsibilities of the professional nurse. The Five Rights of Delegation are: 1) the right task, 2) the right circumstances, 3) the right person, 4) the right direction and communication, and 5) the right supervision and evaluation.

During the last few years, with the changing health care workforce, the decreasing numbers of professional nurses available, and the changing structure of the health care delivery system, more and more unlicensed assistive personnel (UAPs) are functioning in acute care settings. It is imperative that the registered nurse (RN) not only understand his or her own role and responsibilities but also those of the licensed practical nurses (LPNs) and UAPs.

Patient care delivery is increasingly complex. Tasks, including clinical path and outcomes management, are becoming the responsibility of the staff nurse, who needs to learn early on that effective delegation can only help in delivering patient care in a timely manner.

Defining Delegation and Related Concepts

- Nursing delegation is the transfer of authority to perform a designated nursing task to someone who is competent in a particular area. Specific duties need to be delineated clearly.
- All RNs must have a thorough understanding of the scope of practice of all personnel with whom they work. Scope of practice is what the person holding a designated license is legally allowed to perform. For example, an RN is legally able to pronounce a patient expired in a nursing home, whereas this is not within the scope of practice for an LPN.
- Accountability is the taking of legal responsibility for an action.
- Responsibility includes concepts such as reliability, dependability, and obligations to perform professionally.
- Authority is the right—and the official power invested in a position—that an organization gives a designated employee to perform certain tasks.
- The procedure of delegating patient care and duties comes under the assignment-making role of the RN. It is prudent that the RN understands the scope of practice and the competencies of those to whom patient care responsibilities are being delegated.

Responsibilities of the Team Members

- The responsibilities of the nurse manager include ensuring that the correct staffing mix is available on the unit, that competent people are employed, and that enough people are working on a given shift to safely care for the patients.
- The RNs are directly responsible for total patient care delivery. Total care includes patient assessment, diagnosis, planning, implementation, and evaluation. The RN also is responsible for effective delegation and for supervision of LPNs, aides, and other health care team members who may be providing care to patients.
- A new graduate RN has the same accountabilities and responsibilities as a more experienced RN. It is generally understood, however, that new graduates will gradually develop their delegation duties under the mentorship of a more experienced RN.
- In many settings, the LPN has responsibilities similar to those of the RN, except in the areas of patient assessment and certain tasks, such as administering specified medications and taking verbal physician orders.
- The UAPs report either to an LPN or an RN; however, the RN is responsible for the care delivered by the LPNs and the UAPs. The

UAPs can do general direct patient care duties, such as feeding, bathing, ambulation, toileting, and some treatments.

The Five Rights of Delegation

- The Five Rights of Delegation are the right task, under the right circumstance, using the right person, with the right direction and communication and the right supervision.
- A delegation decision-making tree can be found on the website of the National Council of State Boards of Nursing (http://www.ncsbn.org)
- Considerations in delegation are shown in Figure 13-1.

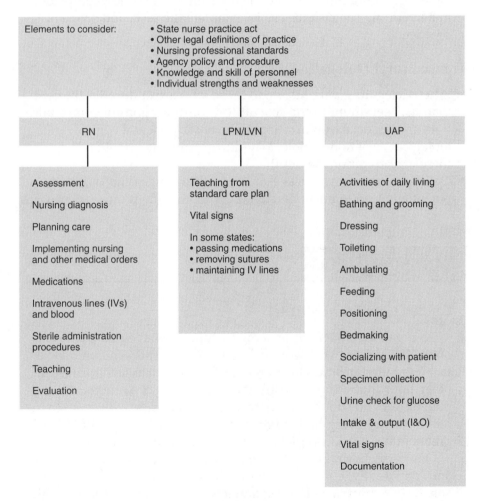

Elements to consider:	• State nurse practice act • Other legal definitions of practice • Nursing professional standards • Agency policy and procedure • Knowledge and skill of personnel • Individual strengths and weaknesses	
RN	**LPN/LVN**	**UAP**
Assessment Nursing diagnosis Planning care Implementing nursing and other medical orders Medications Intravenous lines (IVs) and blood Sterile administration procedures Teaching Evaluation	Teaching from standard care plan Vital signs In some states: • passing medications • removing sutures • maintaining IV lines	Activities of daily living Bathing and grooming Dressing Toileting Ambulating Feeding Positioning Bedmaking Socializing with patient Specimen collection Urine check for glucose Intake & output (I&O) Vital signs Documentation

Figure 13-1   Considerations in Delegation.

Potential Delegation Barriers

- Underdelegation is common in nursing. It may occur when new graduates do not feel they have the skill level or the experience of longer-term employees, or it may occur when managers do not trust the competencies of those they supervise. Generally, underdelegation is a negative behavior, often causing great stress to the person who cannot delegate effectively or appropriately.
- Overdelegation often places the patient at risk, because the person being delegated is often inadequately educated to perform the task or is overwhelmed by too many tasks to complete within a single shift. Again, it is prudent for the person doing the delegating to have a good understanding of a subordinate's abilities, competency in performing the task, desire to complete the task, and scope of practice.

Transcultural Delegation

- When delegating patient care to those who are culturally different than us, keep in mind the six cultural considerations of communication, space, social organization, time, environmental control, and biological variations. Poole, Davidhizar, and Giger (1995) discuss these considerations in depth.
- Cultural differences, unless clearly identified and communicated, potentially lead to misunderstandings about patient care expectations.

CASE SCENARIOS

Guided Case Scenario 13-1

As the RN team leader on a night shift, you have two UAPs and one LPN working with you to care for 20 patients. The unit secretary has called in sick. One of the UAPs is a float assistant from another floor that admits mostly medical oncology patients. All the patients on your floor are general surgery patients, with more than half of them having had surgery that day, and three patients need preoperative work completed before surgery in the morning.

One patient, Mr. Lin, is 4 hours postoperative after back surgery and, apparently, is having complications. He has low blood pressure (80/68; normal is 136/88) and low urinary output (only 20 mL in the last 2 hours). No bed is available in the intensive care unit

(ICU) at the moment, so he needs to be taken care of on the floor until one opens.

Another patient, Ms. Abodo, is also postoperative after abdominal surgery, and she is beginning to hallucinate, is attempting to climb out of bed, and is pulling at her numerous drains and IVs. Her roommate, Ms. Franken, a 92-year-old woman who is two days postoperative for a fractured hip, has dementia and is crying for her father. Their room is across from the dirty utility room toward the end of the hallway so as not to wake all the patients. Ms. Franken needs to begin her 4 units of blood tonight for a low hemoglobin. The remaining patients are mostly stable.

Case Considerations

1. What are some critical factors to consider when deciding what tasks to delegate to the team members?
2. What are some issues in this scenario that may assist you in determining the delegated tasks?
3. Where does one begin when deciding what to delegate and to whom?
4. Identify the tasks that should not be delegated, and why.
5. Are there any legal ramifications to the delegation decisions?
6. Are there any other options to consider?

Case Analysis

1. What are some critical factors to consider when deciding what tasks to delegate to the team members?

   One of the most important things to remember when delegating is that the RN maintains accountability for the decisions regarding what tasks and treatments to delegate. By remembering the Five Rights of Delegation—the right task, the right circumstances, the right person, the right direction and communication, and the right supervision and evaluation— you can then proceed with your decision.

   The RN is accountable not only for her delegation decisions but also responsible for the reliability, dependability, and general obligation to perform nursing care in a competent and acceptable manner. The RN is granted the authority to delegate by the state boards of nursing and nurse practice acts.

   When deciding which tasks to delegate and which to perform yourself, consider the following questions: What tasks are in another person's job description? Do you have personal

knowledge of the person's competency level in performing the
tasks that you would like to delegate? How do you know this?
Have you seen the person's competency check-off forms? Have
you seen the person performing similar tasks in the past?

For the UAP who is floating, pay particular attention to
her skill level to ensure that she is able to perform the tasks
that you delegate to her. Although she is able to take vital
signs, she may not know all the symptoms in postoperative
patients that need to be reported, so clearly review and communicate at the beginning of the shift your expectations
regarding when you need to be notified of significant changes
in patients.

Because the LPN is the only other licensed person on the
unit tonight, you want to review with her any expectations
you may have. In addition, you would probably want to make
sure that she can help to supervise the two UAPs and to
perform any needed treatments.

2. What are some issues in this scenario that may assist in
   determining the delegated tasks?

   Because many of the patients are postoperative, many will
   need frequent vital signs and, probably, pain medication. In
   many states, the LPN cannot administer IV pain medication,
   and any narcotics must be co-signed by an RN. Keeping this
   in mind, take careful note of the patients needing these procedures during your shift.

   Another issue is that of the floating UAP. Although you are
   grateful to the supervisor for the UAP's assistance, you want
   to make sure that she not only is competent in her delegated
   tasks but also is comfortable and feeling supported.

3. Where does one begin in deciding what to delegate and to
   whom?

   The first step in deciding what to delegate is to consider the
   person's job description. What can the person legally do? What
   is outside of the person's scope of practice?

   All patients need a professional nursing assessment, so as
   the RN, you need to ensure that all 20 patients are assessed
   throughout the night. Because frequent vital signs are needed,
   perhaps you want to set up a schedule for both the UAPs, including parameters for when they need to notify you immediately. Can they do intakes and outputs? Can they assist with
   any treatments? Can they assist with ambulation if the patient

has already been out of bed? What tasks can the LPN do to assist you? What care parameters for when to notify you will be given to her?

4. Identify the tasks that should not be delegated, and why.

Again, looking at the person's scope of practice and job description is the most important place to begin. Some tasks and responsibilities clearly are delineated only to the RN. For example, in this state, the LPN cannot administer IV medications, and all narcotics need to be cosigned by an RN.

Mr. Lin's care should not be entirely delegated to the LPN, because it appears that he needs constant assessment of his low blood pressure and UOP. Ms. Adobo is also a potential problem, and although someone cannot sit in her room all night long, she may need to be moved closer to the nursing station.

5. Are there any legal ramifications to the delegation decisions?

The RN must have a clear understanding of the scope of practice for all the personnel she supervises. All RNs are accountable for their decisions. In addition, RNs are legally liable not only for their own actions and decisions in the delegation process but also for the overall nursing care of those patients in their care during a shift. Overdelegation or improper delegation is always a concern, but knowing what the expectations are by the facility and what the legal parameters are according to the state nurse practice act will assist an RN in making informed and appropriate decisions. Planning, clearly communicating expectations, delegating the authority and responsibility needed to complete the tasks, and evaluating patient outcomes are all steps that a prudent RN will take when making decisions regarding delegation.

6. Are there any other options to consider?

The nursing house supervisor may be able to help in several ways. Because a patient who is potentially critically ill is on your floor awaiting an ICU bed, can anyone else be floated temporarily to assist you in taking care of him? Is there, perhaps, a sitter who may be able to stay in Ms. Adobo's room to make sure that she (and her roommate) do not attempt to get out of bed or pull out their drains? Because you do not have a unit secretary, can someone be floated for part of the evening to assist you in taking off orders?

Case Scenario 13-2

Samantha is a new nurse on your unit who has difficulty working with her team members. She is technically competent and makes good decisions, but she insists on doing everything herself. Those tasks that she does delegate, which usually involve vital signs, are always double-checked, giving others a perception that she doesn't trust them—even though most of the staff has been on the unit for more than 10 years. When approached by her manager about her nondelegating style, she simply says, "If you want it done right, you need to do it yourself." You and the others are getting increasingly frustrated and decide to speak with her tonight.

Case Considerations

1. What are some issues that cause you and the staff to speak to Samantha?
2. Why do you think Samantha insists on doing most tasks herself?
3. Discuss how the staff could approach Samantha.
4. What should one not say to Samantha, and why?
5. How can Samantha be helped to understand how effective delegation can benefit both her and the patients?
6. Outline some suggestions for improving Samantha's delegation skills while assisting her in understanding her new role as an RN.

Case Analysis

Samantha is a new RN who does not yet quite know her own limitations and strengths as a leader. When delegating, one runs the risk of either overdelegating or underdelegating to fellow team members. All new graduates feel overwhelmed with the myriad tasks, treatments, assessments, and decisions that they must make by the end of a shift, especially when in nursing school they more than likely didn't have more than a few patients at a time. Even an experienced nurse may occasionally feel overwhelmed by the requirements of caring for patients in an increasingly complex health care system and may not always delegate when indicated.

■ KEY POINTS

1. Delegation is a skill that may be difficult to learn in nursing school, and it may need to be refined while in clinical practice.

2. The RN is always responsible for the care of the patient, regardless of the abilities of the UAPs and LPNs who work with the RN, and is accountable for the delegation of tasks.
3. Often, a new graduate needs guidance in learning the skill of delegation, especially regarding time management and evaluation of the delegated tasks.
4. Many new graduates may feel incompetent and easily overwhelmed, and they may try to "do it all," without asking for help, for fear of appearing to others as a failure. It is the responsibility of the entire health care team to recognize these potential behaviors early in a new nurse's career and to help the nurse understand how effective delegation can actually improve the efficiency of patient care delivery and promote positive patient outcomes.
5. Positive feedback or evaluation of Samantha's growing delegation skills should be offered frequently to help her see how she is progressing.

Case Scenario 13-3

Because of a shortage of RNs, your Vice President of Nursing has decided to place qualified UAPs in the ICU that you manage. He asks you to develop a job description that delineates appropriate tasks that can be delegated by the RN. After consulting with several of your colleagues who already use UAPs in their ICUs, you feel ready to complete your assignment.

Case Considerations

1. Before beginning, review the role of the UAP.
2. What parameters does your state have for the role of the UAP? For the role of the RN who supervises the UAP?
3. Describe the responsibilities of the RN regarding the delegation of patient care tasks to UAPs.
4. Identify 10 tasks or nursing care functions that you would feel comfortable including in the job description for UAPs in the ICU. How does the ICU environment differ from a general medical-surgical floor as far as assigned responsibilities of the UAPs?
5. Identify 10 tasks or nursing care functions that you would not feel comfortable including in the job description for UAPs in the ICU.

Case Analysis

As a cost-saving method, many, if not all, health care systems are using UAPs to augment patient care that is delivered and supervised by the RN. In some agencies, UAPs are hired to replace more expensive licensed personnel, resulting in increased delegation of duties and tasks by the RN. It is imperative that the RN understands the parameters for determining the appropriate use of the UAPs, including job description, demonstrated skills, and competency levels of each person being supervised.

■ KEY POINTS

1. Under no circumstances can UAPs practice nursing or be responsible for the independent delivery of nursing care.
2. UAPs are support personnel who are directly supervised by the RN or, in some situations, an LPN.
3. UAPs cannot assess or evaluate patient responses. Their responsibility is to report these results to the RN.
4. The primary reason for using UAPs is to provide many non-nursing tasks at a lower cost than that with a licensed person.
5. When using UAPs, the scope of practice for an RN is increased.
6. Before assigning a delegated task to a UAP, the RN must assess the individual's skills and knowledge or risk personal liability.

References

Poole, V. L., Davidhizar, R. E., & Giger, J. N. (1995). Delegating to a transcultural team. *Nursing Management, 26* (8), 33–34.

Suggested Readings

Blegan, M. A., Goode, C. J., & Reed, L. (1998). Nurse staffing and patient outcomes. *Nursing Research, 47* (1), 43–50.

Hansten, R. I., & Washburn, M. J.(1998). *Clinical delegation skills* (2nd ed.). Gaithersburg, MD: Aspen Publishers.

Hansten, R. I., & Washburn, M. J. (1998). Why don't nurses delegate? *Journal of Nursing Administration, 26* (12), 24–28.

Hickey, J. V., Ouimette, R. M., & Venegoni, S. L. (1996). *Advanced practice nursing.* Philadelphia: J. B. Lippincott.

Marquis, B. L., & Huston, C. J. (2000). *Leadership roles and management functions* (3rd ed.). Philadelphia: J. B. Lippincott.

Parkman, C. A. (1996). Delegation: Are you doing it right? *American Journal of Nursing, 96* (9), 42–48.

Parsons, L. C. (1998). Delegation skills and nurse job satisfaction. *Nursing Economic$, 16* (1), 18–26.

Pew Health Commission Report. (1995). *Critical challenges: Revitalizing the health professions for the twenty-first century.* San Francisco: USCF Center for Health Professions.

Managing Care

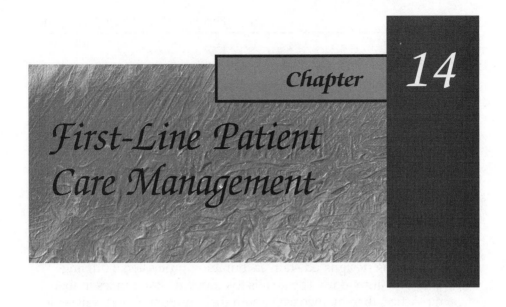

Chapter

14

First-Line Patient Care Management

Essential Concepts in Patient Care Management

One of the pivotal positions in the health care system is the first-line manager. The first-line manager communicates directly with and coordinates the messages of many people, including patients and their families, nursing and other staff members, physicians, and administrators. Skills such as expert communication, negotiation, active listening, and multitasking are valued in the first-line manager, because this role interacts and makes decisions for a wide variety of people and situations.

Essential to the success of patient care is the effective application of strategic unit planning, developing a structure and a process for professional practice, and ensuring competency in the staff. Each of these steps requires the first-line manager's involvement and input. The first-line manager should be able to manage and to lead staff, achieving results through his or her vision for unit improvement.

First-Line Management Defined

- By applying the nursing process, first-line management plans, implements, and evaluates the care of a specific patient population that is geographically situated.

Strategic Planning

- Strategic planning is the process of delineating goals and objectives within a specified period of time.
- In developing a strategic plan, the first phase is an assessment of the external and internal environments.
- Next, the philosophy, mission, and vision statements should be reviewed for congruence and to clarify the institution's values and beliefs.

Shared Governance Concepts

- In a shared governance environment, leadership is decentralized and shared among designated staff, encouraging professional nursing practice and autonomy. The goal is to empower staff nurses in their own practice, thereby increasing both their autonomy and satisfaction.
- Shared governance is most successful when the entire organization practices this model.
- Common components of a shared governance model (Figure 14-1) include a clinical practice council, a quality council, an education council, a research council, a management council, and possibly, a coordinating council.

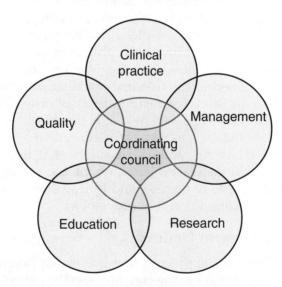

Shared Goverance Model

Figure 14-1 A Shared Governance Model.

- The functions of the various councils are to promote staff nurse responsibility and accountability for professional nursing care, decreasing the role of the centralized model of management.
- The role of the nurse manager in a shared governance environment becomes more consultative, collaborative, and mentoring rather than directive. Often, the cost and length of time that would be needed to successfully introduce and maintain this type of model outweighs its many benefits.

Benner's Novice to Expert Theory

- The Novice to Expert Theory of Benner (1984) identifies five stages of progressive skill acquisition for nurses and is based on the theoretical work of Dreyfus and Dreyfus (1980).
- New graduate nurses fall into the novice stage, in which they are predominately task- and skill-oriented. Advanced beginners demonstrate some independent thinking and decision-making once task competency is established. A competent nurse has been functioning in his or her role for 2 to 3 years, has grown comfortable with longer-range planning activities, and has greater performance efficiency.
- Professional proficient nurses draw on experiences to help them devise a total patient care plan; their own experiences help them to know what the potential outcomes are given in certain data sets. Finally, the true expert nurse is one who relies not only on experiences but also on a sense of intuition to make patient care decisions.
- First-line managers will work with staff members at all levels of Benner's model.

Accountability-Based Care Delivery

- Accountability-based care delivery includes the primary care, the patient-focused care, and the case management models to achieve quality patient outcomes.

CASE SCENARIOS

Guided Case Scenario 14-1

The clinical ladder model at your institution is scheduled for review, and you have been asked to lead the committee. The institution currently has two levels: professional nurse, which is BSN only; and nonprofessional nurse, which includes registered nurses (RNs) with diploma and associate degree preparation. The licensed practical nurses (LPNs) are not included on the ladder; however, the staff mix at the institution contains 28% LPNs. The BSN-prepared nurses acknowledge that they appreciate differentiating between the two levels. They only receive a 2% differential in pay and no other additional benefits, yet they must provide at least four in-services a year, act as charge nurses, and attend one outside conference each year, for which they pay 25% of the total costs. The BSN nurses are generally unhappy with the present clinical ladder. The non-BSN nurses say they have no incentive to continue their education and are content with the current situation, whereas the BSN nurses are increasingly vocal about their unhappiness with the clinical ladder.

Case Considerations

1. Describe the purpose of a clinical ladder in a health care institution.
2. Who should be included on the committee to review the clinical ladder model, and why?
3. Identify some of the current issues that the committee needs to address as it looks to revise the clinical ladder.
4. Which nursing theorist would provide a framework for the committee to redesign their clinical ladder, and why?
5. Discuss a tentative outline for the new clinical ladder model that your committee would propose.

Case Analysis

1. Describe the purpose of a clinical ladder in a health care institution.

   The purpose of a clinical ladder in a health care system is to acknowledge a nurse's professional practice and education through a human resources—driven reward and recognition system. All nurses begin at designated points on the "ladder," depending on education, experience, certifications, and other predetermined factors, and they "move up the ladder" when certain expectations are met. A clinical ladder promotes skill and professional development in the professional nursing ranks by differentiating between nurses and their accomplishments while focusing on clinical and managerial competency.

The first-line manager is responsible for the development of professional staff and for reviewing the costs versus the recruiting and retention points of maintaining the clinical ladder system. Many professional staff value a clinical ladder system for promotion and retention, because it clearly identifies and rewards those nurses who are active within the organization and who maintain practice competency.

2. Who should be included on the committee to review the clinical ladder model, and why?

The first thing to do in putting together a committee to review the current clinical ladder structure is to consider who it affects as well as who the revised clinical ladder could affect. The scenario states that the current ladder divides nurses into two sections: those that are BSN-prepared, and those that are not. To ensure an equal voice, the committee should have both groups represented along with nurses who have reached higher degrees (e.g., those who are Masters-prepared). To round out the committee, include nonnurses, who may be able to identify issues that could potentially affect the hospital, plus managers, an administrator (e.g., the Vice President for Nursing), and someone who represents the Human Resources Department.

3. Identify some of the current issues that the committee needs to address as it looks to revise the clinical ladder.

Several concerns about the current clinical ladder situation require attention:

a. The issue of dividing the clinical ladder into BSN-prepared nurses and non-BSN-prepared nurses.

b. The issue of BSN-prepared nurses only receiving a 2% differential in pay for having a degree.

c. The issue of increased responsibility and expectations for having a BSN while receiving only a 2% differential in pay.

d. The current ladder only having two levels and not taking into account graduate preparation or those who are actively pursuing degrees.

e. General dissatisfaction about the clinical ladder, which will take some work by the committee to re-engage the staff.

f. Lack of incentive for the non-BSN-prepared nurses to continue their education.

4. Which nursing theorist would provide a framework for the committee to redesign their clinical ladder, and why?

Patricia Benner (1984) is a popular nursing theorist, and her Novice to Expert Theory has been applied by many health care institutions to the clinical ladder concept. This theory expounds on the expanding skill sets that a nurse accomplishes as he or she progresses in experience, both in years and in situations. This particular model works well as a framework for a clinical ladder model, because it explains that as a nurse acquires more experience over the course of a career, that nurse is also developing new skills and refining those already acquired. There are five stages to role development in the Novice to Expert Theory: novice, advanced beginner, competent, proficient, and expert. Benner states that nurses move from the task-oriented novice stage through competency to the delivery of expert, intuitive care to their clients.

5. Discuss a tentative outline for the new clinical ladder model that your committee would propose.

A tentative outline would be:

a. Develop a focus group to review the current clinical ladder for its advantages and disadvantages. This group needs to keep in mind the concerns outlined in answer 2 and to make recommendations to the task force.

b. Once the committee has reviewed the focus group's recommendations, perform a survey of clinical ladders at other institutions to identify key aspects of models that your facility may like to include in its new model.

c. Decide on a framework. Does the committee wish to model after the Novice to Expert Theory of Benner?

d. Decide who should be included in the clinical ladder. Should only RNs be included, or should the LPNs be included as well?

e. Outline the levels of the ladder. What is included on each level, and what is needed for promotion? What will be included in a portfolio? Who is responsible for reviewing the portfolios?

f. Work with the Human Resources Department to review the compensation for not only BSN-prepared nurses but also for anyone who climbs the ladder.

g. Finally, there needs to be a distinct role for the nurse manager in the clinical ladder process. The committee can recommend to the Vice President for Nursing and the Human Resources Department potential responsibilities and functions for a nurse manager and still maintain the shared governance focus.

Case Scenario 14-2

Your nurse manager has asked you to assist her in transitioning the three intensive care units (ICUs) into shared governance models. The new Vice President for Nursing is a strong proponent of professional nursing and believes that nurses will have more job satisfaction when they become more actively involved with the management and leadership of their unit. Currently, all the staff are RNs who practice primary nursing, but there is talk about hiring unlicensed assistive personnel (UAPs) into the ICUs because of the nursing shortage.

Case Considerations

1. What is shared governance? How is this model different from the primary care nursing model?
2. Identify five councils that commonly comprise the shared governance model and their purposes. Are any other councils appropriate to add?
3. What do you believe the Vice President for Nursing hopes to accomplish with implementation of the shared governance model?

Case Analysis

The shared governance model is popular in institutions where the staffing pattern includes many professional nurses. For the shared governance model to be implemented effectively, nursing leadership needs to hold the belief that clinicians and managers can work well together to accomplish optimal decision-making.

▪ KEY POINTS

1. The shared governance model is based on decentralized leadership strategies.
2. Autonomous decision-making is valued, along with collaborative problem solving.
3. Having staff actively participate in the councils enables nurses to realize fully their professional practice.
4. Shared governance models empower nurses to have more control over their practice.

5. There has to be a clearly identified role for the nurse manager within the shared governance model.

References

Benner, P. (1984). *From novice to expert*. Menlo Park, CA: Addison-Wesley.

Dreyfus, S. E., & Dreyfus, H. L. (1980). *A five stage model of the mental activities involved with skill acquisition*. Unpublished report supported by the USAF (Contract F49620-79-C-0063), University of California at Berkeley.

Suggested Readings

Blegan, M. A., Goode, C. J., & Reed, L. (1998). Nurse staffing and patient outcomes. *Nursing Research, 47* (1), 43–50.

Dirschel, K. M. (1994). Decentralization or centralization: Striking a balance. *Nursing Management, 25* (9), 49–51.

Hess, R. G., Jr. (1995). Shared governance: Nursing's 20th century tower of Babel. *Journal of Nursing Administration, 25* (5), 14–17.

Hickey, J. V., Ouimette, R. M., & Venegoni, S. L. (1996). *Advanced practice nursing*. Philadelphia: J. B. Lippincott.

Lacshinger, H. K., & Havens, D. S. (1996). Staff nurse work empowerment and perceived control over nursing practice. *Journal of Nursing Administration, 26* (9), 27–35.

Marquis, B. L., & Huston, C. J. (2000). *Leadership roles and management functions* (3rd ed.). Philadelphia: J. B. Lippincott.

Martin, M. (1998). Achieving the right balance with strategic planning. *Nursing Management, 29* (5), 30–31.

Neubauer, J. (1997). Beyond hierarchy: Working on the edge of chaos. *Journal of Nursing Management, 5* (2), 65–67.

Porter O'Grady, T. (1992). *Implementing shared governance: Creating a professional organization*. St. Louis, MO: Mosby–Year Book.

Truscott, J. P., & Churchill, G. M. (1998). Patient focused care: Improving customer satisfaction while reducing costs. In E. C. Hein (Ed.), *Contemporary leadership behavior*. Philadelphia: Lippincott-Raven.

Vestal, K. W., Fralic, R. D., & Spreier, S. W. (1997). Organizational culture: The link between strategy and results. *Hospital and Health Services Administration, 42* (3), 339–365.

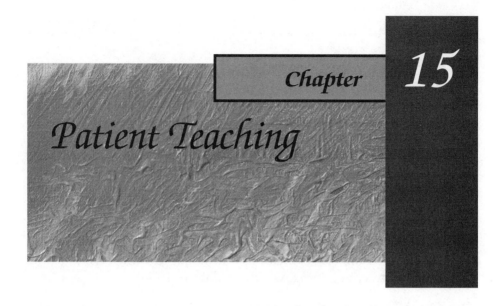

Chapter 15

Patient Teaching

Essential Concepts in Patient Teaching

Teaching patients and their families is an inherent role of the professional nurse and is closely woven into everyday practice. Teaching enhances nursing care. It promotes a patient's independence with informed decision-making about their health care. Today, much health care information is available to the public, especially on the Internet and in the media, than ever before. It is also the responsibility of the registered nurse to assist the patient in discriminating between actual health information and that information which is clearly false, misleading, and will cause incorrect health care decisions. Having a more informed patient will usually result in enhanced patient care outcomes and reduced health care costs, not only to the institution but to the family as well.

Major Steps of a Teaching Methodology

- The five primary steps of a teaching methodology are analysis, design, development, implementation, and evaluation.

The Analysis Phase of Teaching

- To establish what type of teaching is needed, a nurse needs to review the situational context in which the teaching will occur: when, where, and why that teaching is necessary.
- A learner analysis, which is a process for developing an individualized teaching plan, is performed. An individual's demographic background and learning styles are key areas to consider when devising a teaching-learning plan.
- Everyone learns using different learning techniques and styles. Three predominant learning styles and their theories include perceptive learning, information processing, and personality traits. The theory of Kolb (1984) includes four major learning styles: sensing, abstracting, doing, watching (Figure 15-1).

The Three Domains of Learning

- The last component in the analysis phase of teaching is to determine what content actually is to be taught based on the three learning domains: cognitive, psychomotor, and affective. Not all content lends itself to all domains, and the nurse must assess which method(s) will best teach the patient. The learning domains have a hierarchy of behaviors.
- The cognitive domain focuses on what the learner actually understands as knowledge (Bloom & Krathwohl, 1956).
- The psychomotor domain is skill focused and uses the five senses to learn about a particular concept (Simpson, 1971).
- In the affective domain, feelings, values, and beliefs are the focus, with the nurse assisting the learner to understand his or her attitudes toward a particular topic (Krathwohl, Bloom, & Masia, 1999).
- For example, patients may cognitively understand why they have to administer insulin to themselves and be physically able to administer the insulin. However, these patients may have difficulty accepting that they need insulin to maintain their health.

Developing Behavioral Objectives

- Behavioral objectives identify what the learner is expected to achieve at the completion of the teaching—in other words, the measurable outcome.
- The four components of a behavioral objective are the audience or performer, the performance needed to achieve the outcome, the degree of meeting the expectation, and the conditions placed on the performance.

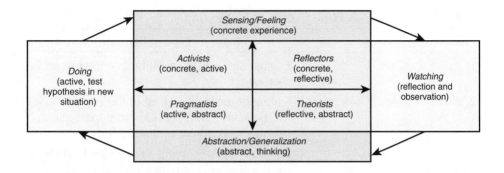

Type	Combinations
Activists	Sensing/feeling: Perceive information in concrete rather than theoretical ways; peer-oriented, social
	Doing: look for practical, physical applications of learning
Reflectors	Sensing/feeling: Perceive information in concrete rather than theoretical ways; peer-oriented, social
	Watching: Want to observe, reflect, and establish objective interpretations of information;judge own performance by external, objective measures rather than personal, subjective judgment.
Theorists	Watching: Want to observe, reflect, and establish objective interpretations of information; judge own performance by external, objective measures rather than personal, subjective judgment.
	Abstraction/generalization: Prefer theory and systematic analysis; want structured learning experience; more oriented toward things, less toward people.
Pragmatists	Doing: look for practical, physical applications of learning
	Abstraction/generalization: Prefer theory and systematic analysis; want structured learning experience; more oriented toward things, less toward people.

Figure 15-1   Kolb's Experiential Learning Style. Compiled from Kolb (1984).

Terminal and Enabling Objectives

- A terminal objective is a major behavior that, once completed successfully, adds to the learner's goal.
- An enabling objective offers support in meeting the terminal objectives and is often a secondary behavior that assists the learner with achieving the overall goal.

Gagne's Key Learning Events

- To facilitate the learning process, applying Gagne's (1985) nine events of instruction is helpful in conducting the learning session (Table 15-1).

Table 15-1   Gagne's Nine Events of Instruction

Event	Explanation
1. Gain attention.	Engage the learner and stimulate interest and motivation.
2. Inform learner of objective.	Stating objectives establishes the expectations for the learner and provides an opportunity to preview the content of the teaching event.
3. Stimulate recall of prerequisite learning.	Try to relate the content to previous learning or experience. This provides the learner with a familiar context in which to approach learning.
4. Present stimulus materials.	Present the content.
5. Provide learning guidance.	Perform/demonstrate the learning for the learner or in conjunction with the learner.
6. Elicit performance.	Have the learner practice or demonstrate the learning.
7. Provide feedback.	Help the learner refine learning by providing feedback and suggestions.
8. Assess performance.	Evaluate learner performance in terms of the learning objectives.
9. Enhance retention and transfer.	Review learning and encourage learner to use learning in new situations.

Compiled from Gagne (1985).

- According to Gagne (1985), the nine key events range from gaining the attention of the learner to providing the teaching materials and, in the process of evaluating the knowledge gained, enhancing retention and transfer of the new information.

Evaluation of Teaching

- When evaluating the teaching session, either the teacher is being evaluated for his or her effectiveness in sharing knowledge or the learner is being evaluated for the knowledge gained.
- The goal of the learner evaluation is to determine if the objectives of the teaching session were met. The learner evaluation can include methods such as recall, demonstration, test taking, or problem solving in a given scenario.
- The goal of the teaching evaluation is to determine the effectiveness of the teaching session and of the teacher and look for ways to improve on the teaching process. Feedback is sought using a variety of methods, including verbal discussions and written evaluations.

CASE SCENARIOS

Guided Case Scenario 15-1

Congratulations! As the most senior clinical nurse on the medical endocrinology floor, you have been selected to become the diabetic nurse educator. The floor has not had anyone functioning in this role for more than 10 years, and the diabetic materials available for both the patients and the nurses are more than 8 years old.

As you sit with your manager, he states his confidence that you will be able to develop three separate diabetic teaching programs: a program for the patients, a program for the professional staff, and a program for the public. Never having taught formally, you immediately sign up for a graduate course on teaching theory at the local university.

Case Considerations

1. Where does one begin? What resources can be used?
2. How will the three programs differ? Do the three programs need to be different?
3. All standard teaching methodologies have five major phases. What are these phases, and what specifics do the phases contain?
4. Design a learning goal for each of the three programs.
5. Identify the three taxonomies of learning, and give one example of each as it applies to diabetic self-care activities.
6. How should one evaluate success in each of the three programs?

Case Analysis

1. Where does one begin? What resources can be used?

The first step is to see if the hospital has any other educators so that you can meet them and, perhaps, ask them to mentor you. It is always easier to work with someone who has already-established programs in place. Sometimes, however, just finding available rooms in an institution is an undertaking!

Because this is your first position as an educator and 10 years have passed since the last formal position, the learners need to be identified and their specific characteristics analyzed. Perform a needs survey for all three groups, because each group has unique learning and content needs. If your institution has other educators, perhaps they have needs surveys already developed that you can adapt for diabetes teaching.

Once you understand the needs of each population, it is time to obtain resources. Besides the resources found in the institution, such as the medical library, you may want to look to community and, perhaps, even national resources for information. Many national organizations even have booklets, handouts, and videos that can be purchased in bulk, saving you countless hours in creating materials. Do speakers in the community have expertise in the area of diabetes? If so, you may want to contact them as well. You will need to work closely with your manager to ensure that any materials needed will be included in a budgetary request.

2. How will the three programs differ? Do the three programs need to be different?

Each of the three populations—patients, professional staff, and the public—have different needs and learning styles. Some materials may be appropriate for all three, such as a listing of community and national resources, whereas other materials will have to be altered for the specific audience. If you are teaching about the pathophysiology behind diabetes, the public will need the most basic information, a patient more, and a professional the most in-depth information.

The patient population will contain some who have been newly diagnosed, both with type I and type II diabetes, who will need similar information. Those with type I diabetes will also require information on insulin injection information and skill acquisition. In addition, you will be called on to teach those patients with diabetes that may be uncontrolled for a variety of reasons, including lifestyle, diet, and improper medication administration, so individual teaching plans will need to be developed.

Professional staff should already understand the basic pathophysiology behind diabetes, medication administration, and dietary considerations. What this population will need are updates to the above content, perhaps a periodic review of the different medications and administration methods, plus information on blood sugar–testing techniques. Some states also require continuing education, so there may be an opportunity to develop some of these programs for credit.

The public may want a general introduction to the topic of diabetes and be more interested in screening for rather than actually learning about the disease. Public sessions are a wonderful way to introduce people to the services that a health care system offers, so information on both inpatient and outpatient services is important to include.

3. All standard teaching methodologies have five major phases. What are these phases, and what specifics do the phases contain?

   The five steps to developing a teaching plan include analysis, design, development, implementation, and evaluation—much like the nursing process. In the analysis phase, the educator discovers what type of learning is needed and examines context, learner types, and content. In the design phase, learning goals and objectives are established, and measurable outcomes are defined. Deciding what content to teach and how to teach it occurs during the development stage. The format for the learning sessions is outlined, with the educator deciding on the most appropriate media and presentation materials to reach the learning goals. During the implementation stage, the actual teaching occurs. After the teaching session ends, the educator should always review the effectiveness of the session, using the viewpoints of both the educator and the learner in evaluating whether goals and objectives were met. Evaluation can be in the form of a verbal review, a written review, or even a skills demonstration, but regardless of the methodology, an evaluation process should be performed to ascertain whether the correct message was sent.

4. Design a learning goal for each of the three programs.

   Learning goal for the patient session: At the completion of the learning session, the patient will be able to accurately perform diabetic self-care techniques.

   Learning goal for the professional staff session: At the completion of the learning session, the professional staff nurse will be able to differentiate between the types of insulin available for patient use by describing the actions, properties, administration, and side effects of each.

   Learning goal for the public session: At the completion of the learning session, the community member will be able to identify the hallmark signs and symptoms of diabetes mellitus.

5. Identify the three taxonomies of learning, and give one example of each as it applies to diabetic self-care activities.

There are three taxonomies of learning: cognitive (Bloom & Krathwohl, 1956), affective (Krathwohl et al., 1999), and psychomotor (Simpson, 1971). In the cognitive domain, the educator evaluates the learner's acquired knowledge regarding a topic, such as whether the patient can identify the signs and symptoms of foot neuropathy as a result of poor foot care. With the affective domain, the patient is asked to describe how he or she feels about a certain aspect of the content. Does the patient accept the need to take extra cautions about self-care and their feet, or do they ignore a cut on the foot, saying that it will heal in time? Finally, the psychomotor phase requires a demonstration of skill attainment for mastery of the content. With the psychomotor phase, the nurse may observe the patient correctly providing self-foot care, such as cutting nails.

6. How should one evaluate success in each of the three programs?

The content of each program may be drastically different, but it is always important to evaluate whether the educator presented the material in a manner that enabled learning— and whether learning actually occurred during the session. The objectives and goals will guide the educator in determining what content to evaluate. It does not matter what the content is or how simple or how complex the topic; the process of evaluation enables the educator to determine whether the teaching was effective. Evaluation also offers insight regarding how to improve the presentation of material. Areas to consider in the evaluation process include patient learning, patient satisfaction, the environment in which the session occurred, the relevance of the topic and the content, the pacing of the session, and the delivery style of the educator in presenting the information.

Case Scenario 15-2

As a senior-level nursing student, one of your classes is Community Health. One of the assigned projects is to develop a teaching session for hypertension based on the nine events of instruction according to Gagne (1985).

Case Considerations

1. Outline the nine events of instruction, giving a brief explanation for each event.
2. Develop a teaching plan for the prevention of hypertension based on this framework.
3. Why is Gagne's work helpful in planning the teaching session?
4. During the development stage of the teaching process, several other techniques should be kept in mind while planning the teaching session. What are these other techniques, and how should they be used in the development phase?

Case Analysis

Sometimes, the most detailed lesson plan turns into a disastrous teaching session when resources are not carefully considered during the development phase. Issues such as format, strategies, appropriate media resources, and lesson plans assist the educator in ensuring that the final teaching session is presented in a comprehensive manner.

▌ KEY POINTS

1. During the development phase of planning the teaching session, presentation format, media, strategies for teaching, and the lesson plan are considered.
2. The nine events of instruction is helpful to the educator in providing guidelines and as a suggested structure for an effective learning session.
3. The types of strategies considered in the teaching plan are often determined by the learner's needs and style of learning.
4. Many teaching sessions, although containing excellent content, often are not seen as effective as they could be because of the types of materials and media that have been selected to get the message across to the recipient.
5. A lesson plan assists the educator in providing a road map for the teaching session. A well-developed lesson plan allows another educator to teach the same information, using the same blueprint, with hopefully the same results.

Case Scenario 15-3

One of the biggest challenges is teaching pediatric patients who are newly diagnosed with diabetes and who often require frequent blood testing as the providers attempt to regulate their insulin administrations. Today, you face a huge challenge in Nick, a 13-year-old Hispanic male who is obese. Nick was diagnosed with juvenile diabetes a year ago. Today, he is admitted onto the floor with a blood sugar of 624 after a weekend visit to his dad's house. According to the admitting physician's notes, Nick's blood sugar has been largely uncontrolled for the entire year. Nick admits to you that "It's not cool to stick myself with needles." He also says, "I only check my sugars once in awhile." The physician orders diabetic teaching for Nick—one more time.

Case Considerations

1. What are some issues to consider immediately when dealing with Nick?
2. What are the top five priorities, in decreasing order, of teaching Nick? Why are they ranked in this order?
3. What can one assume are some of the issues important to Nick, and why?
4. What type of teaching sessions should one develop?
5. Identify the content of the teaching sessions.
6. Design four behavioral objectives for the teaching sessions.
7. How should one evaluate success in presenting the teaching sessions?

Case Analysis

Every learner has his or her own needs and style of learning, and it is important for the nurse educator to have at least a basic understanding of both before planning a teaching session. Complicating this particular teaching session is the fact that the educator is working with a teenager who not only has a chronic disease needing constant attention but is also dealing with normal developmental issues and may need a variety of teaching methodologies for a positive outcome.

■ KEY POINTS

1. One of the first steps to perform is a learner analysis: Nick has had his disease for more than a year. However, his diabetes is still uncontrolled, and he is apparently dealing with some issues surrounding the disease.

2. Demographics are important data sets to keep in mind when planning a teaching session. In Nick's case, he is a young male, obese, and of Hispanic descent. Any and all of these demographics may be contributing to his unwillingness to learn and to apply his knowledge to his disease.
3. Learning styles are the ways in which people learn best. Some learners are tactile. Some are auditory. Some prefer reading about the information first. Learning styles assist the educator in deciding on the appropriate teaching strategies for the client.
4. Sometimes, it is helpful to provide support for the learner through others. In Nick's case, other children who have diabetes—and have successfully lived with the disease—may be good resources for him.
5. Mutual goal setting is one method to apply when dealing with a learner who is resistant to acquiring new knowledge or to applying already learned information. In mutual goal setting, the nurse could establish a contract with Nick for his learning: Perhaps what he wants to learn is much different from what the nurse perceives his needs to be.

References

Bloom, B. S., & Krathwohl, D. (1956). *Taxonomy of educational objectives: Handbook I: Cognitive domain.* Boston: Addison-Wesley.

Gagne, R. M. (1985). *The conditions of learning and the history of instruction* (4th ed.). New York: Holt, Rinehart, & Winston.

Kolb, D. A. (1984). *Experiential learning: Experience as the source of learning and development.* Englewood Cliffs, NJ: Prentice-Hall/TPR.

Krathwohl, D. R., Bloom, B. S., & Masia, B. B. (1999). *Taxonomy of educational objectives: Handbook 2I: Affective domain.* Boston: Addison-Wesley.

Simpson, E. (1971). Educational objectives in the psychomotor domain. In M. Kapfer (Ed.), *Behavioral objectives in curriculum development.* Englewood Cliffs, NJ: Educational Technology.

Suggested Readings

Ballentine, L. (2003). On education. Games as an education and retention strategy. *CANNT Journal, 13* (1), 46–48.

Belar, C. (2003). Speaking of education: Competencies for quality health care. *American Psychological Association.* 34, no. 7.

Benner, P. (1984). *From novice to expert.* Menlo Park, CA: Addison-Wesley.

Bruccoliere, T. (2000). How to make patient teaching stick. *RN, 63* (2), 34–38.

Hickey, J. V., Ouimette, R. M., & Venegoni, S. L. (1996). *Advanced practice nursing.* Philadelphia: J. B. Lippincott.

Learmonth, A., & Watson, N. (1999). Constructing evidence based health promotion: Perspectives from the field. *Critical Public Health, 19,* 317–333.

MacLeod-Clark, J., & Maben, J. (1999). Health promotion in primary health care nursing: the development of quality indicators. *Health Education Journal, 58,* 99–119.

Whitehead, D. (2003). Evaluating health promotion: A model for nursing practice. *Journal of Advanced Nursing, 41* (5), 490–498.

Chapter 16

Change and Conflict Resolution

Essential Concepts in Change and Conflict Resolution

Situations of change and conflict predictably arise regardless of where one is employed, especially when there are numerous influences both inside and outside of the health care organization. The prudent manager, however, has the responsibility to guide staff through these changing situations, helping them to understand the factors leading to the change and requesting input as decisions are made to plan, implement, and evaluate the process of change.

When a change occurs in the balance of a situation, there is a possibility that a difference in opinions will occur, which could result in a conflict among people. Once, all conflict was thought to be a sign of an unhealthy work environment. Today, theorists realize that some conflict not only is inevitable but also can promote growth and understanding where it did not exist before the conflict situation. Regardless of the setting, the staff nurse needs to develop solid conflict management and resolution skills to work with patients and coworkers alike.

Change Perspectives

- Change can occur at several different levels. Personal change is made for the individual and is generally brought on by a need for self-improvement. Professional change often occurs when a different position is sought, additional education is earned, or different opportunities are desired. Organizational change is often initiated to improve a process or outcomes at the organizational level and, like all change, is generally planned.

Change Theorists

- The Force Field Model of Lewin (1951) is often used to illustrate how planned change can occur. This model includes three steps: unfreezing, movement, and refreezing. The force field analysis component reviews the positive reasons for the change and compares them to the negative reasons inhibiting the change. When the reasons for not keeping the changes equal the reasons for making the change, there is equilibrium. Only when there is disequilibrium in the system will change occur.
- Lewin's model influenced several other theorists, including Lippit, Watson, and Westley (1958). In the Phases of Change Theory, those authors identify seven stages in the process of change: (1) diagnosis of the problem, (2) assessment of the motivation for change and the capacity of the person to change, (3) assessment of the change agent's motivation for change and his or her capacity to change, (4) accurate selection of the change objectives, (5) choosing an appropriate role for the change agent, (6) maintaining the change once it has been initiated, (7) and ending the relationship between the change agent and those changed.
- Havelock (1973) also expanded on Lewin's original theory, including more steps in each of the three phases. Havelock focuses on the planning phase, during which he believes many who act as change agents need to place more emphasis on to ensure a smooth change process.
- Rogers (1983) uses Lewin's Force Field Model as a basis for his Diffusion of Innovations Theory, which holds that change can be initiated, stopped, and readopted at another point in time. Rogers emphasizes how change often does not have an even course: There may be many stops and starts until the end objective is met successfully.

The Learning Organization

- An organization, by its nature, is an open system. A learning organization is one that, in its attempt to initiate, maintain, and evaluate

change, is flexible and responsive, looking constantly for ways to improve financial, personnel, and patient outcomes.
- Senge (1990) identifies five disciplines that he believes are critical to the development of the learning organization: systems thinking, personal mastery, mental models, building shared vision, and team learning.

Change Strategies

- To find a method that can be used to initiate change, the nursing process can be applied. When applying the change process to the nursing process, the steps would be assessment, planning, implementation of the change strategies, evaluation of the change, and an added phase, stabilization of the change. It is important to assess the effect of the change and whether the change has now become the norm.
- Bennis, Benne, and Chinn (1969) identified three primary strategies for effecting change in others. First, in applying the notion of rational-empirical strategy, evidence is given in the form of current research in the belief that humans are rational beings who, to make a change, need to see the documented evidence first. Second, those who are more group thinkers would participate in change that is normative-reductive or that uses group norms to influence decisions. Third, those who employ authority, political clout, or simply their influence to make a change are using power-coercive strategies.

The Role of the Change Agent

- A change agent is the person who leads the change process. The change agent may or may not be part of the organization.
- The most crucial responsibilities of the change agent include keeping the channels of communication open, keeping the momentum for change moving in a positive direction, and expressing enthusiasm for the change project even when problems occur.
- In the planning process, an effective change agent includes those people who are affected by the proposed change, encouraging ownership and valuing their input.
- When the change is complete, it is time to switch ownership of the process from the change agent to those who will maintain the change.

Conflict

- Conflict is either internal or external, real or perceived differences either within a person or among people.

- Conflict can be categorized into three broad areas: intrapersonal, interpersonal, and organizational or intergroup.
- Sources of conflict are differences in ideas, values, beliefs or feelings, threats that are both internal and external, resource allocations, personalities, and competitions.

The Conflict Process

- Filley (1975) suggests that there are five steps to the conflict process: antecedent conditions, perceived and/or felt conflict, manifest behavior, conflict resolution or suppression, and resolution aftermath. Filley believes that both conflict and conflict resolution follow a specific process, going through these five stages sequentially.
- Not all conflict scenarios are handled in the same manner, especially if resolution of the conflict is the ultimate goal. At least seven techniques for conflict resolution are currently accepted (Table 16-1). These methods to assist those in conflict are avoidance, accommodation, competing, compromising, negotiation, collaboration, and confronting. The goal should always be a win-win situation— in other words, a situation in which both parties are comfortable with the results and neither has had to compromise their values to achieve the goal. Clear communication always facilitates the dissolution of conflict.

CASE SCENARIOS

Guided Case Scenario 16-1

The hospital where you are employed just instituted a clinical ladder program, in which educational advancement is rewarded not only monetarily but also with a preferred staffing pattern and fewer rotations. As an upgrade to the benefits package, tuition benefits are also increased for full-time employees. As a parent of three children under 3 years of age, you find it increasingly difficult to locate a sitter during the off-shift to bridge the gap between when you leave for work and when your spouse (who is also on shift work) arrives home.

As a BSN-prepared nurse, you have always wanted to go back to graduate school to become a clinical nurse specialist. Is now the right time to go back to school?

Table 16-1   Summary of Conflict Resolution Techniques

Conflict Resolution Technique	Advantages	Disadvantages
Avoiding—ignoring the conflict	Does not make a big deal out of nothing; conflict may be minor in comparison to other priorities	Conflict can become bigger than antici- pated; source of con- flict might be more important to one person or group than others
Accommodating— smoothing or cooperating. One side gives in to the other side	One side is more con- cerned with an issue than the other side; stakes not high enough for one group and that side is willing to give in	One side holds more power and can force the other side to give in; the importance of the stakes are not as apparent to one side as the other; can lead to parties feeling "used" if they are always pressured to give in
Competing—forcing; the two or three sides are forced to compete for the goal	Produces a winner; good when time is short and stakes are high	Produces a loser; leaves anger and resentment on losing sides
Compromising—each side gives up something and gains something	No one should win or lose but both should gain something; good for disagreements between individuals	May cause a return to the conflict if what is given up becomes more important than the original goal
Negotiating—high-level discussion that seeks agreement but not necessarily consensus	Stakes are very high and solution is rather per- manent; often involves powerful groups	Agreements are per- manent, even though each side has gains and losses
Collaborating—both sides work together to develop optimal outcome	Best solution for the con- flict and encompasses all important goals to each side	Takes a lot of time; requires commitment to success
Confronting—immediate and obvious movement to stop conflict at the very start	Does not allow conflict to take root; very powerful	May leave impression that conflict is not tolerated; may make something big out of nothing

Case Considerations

1. What are the issues, and why is there a conflict?
2. Applying Lewin's Force Field Model, identify three positives for returning to school now and three negatives for going back to school now.
3. Are there any alternative solutions to this situation?
4. What would be an implementation schedule for the desired change?

Case Analysis

1. What are the issues, and why is there a conflict?

   Returning to school is a dream that many people have, yet it often remains an unfulfilled dream because of other obligations and unplanned issues. Whether to return to graduate school is not the issue at hand. The issue is whether this is the best time to return to school when all the circumstances are considered.

   The institution just implemented a wonderful clinical ladder, in which increased education is rewarded. With a bachelor's degree in nursing, you have already been placed on the second "rung" of the ladder, above those with more tenure but without a 4-year college degree. With a master's degree in nursing, you could be placed on the fifth rung of the ladder, at the top. There is also the potential for a $30,000 difference in salary on the day shift. You would have increased demands made on your time by attending school and adding the schoolwork to your already busy schedule. Graduate school is something that you have always known you would complete, and it is just a matter of going now rather than later. You not only have the desire, but you have the drive to accomplish this goal.

   The complications, or conflict, are the more critical issues of family, finances, and time not only to work but also to study. It is not an easy task to perform shift work and also raise three small children, but staying at home is not an option financially for your family. You enjoy working in the hospital, and you can see yourself working there for many years. However, to be promoted and taken off the rotating schedule, you need to return to school to earn a higher degree—hence the conflict.

2. Applying Lewin's Force Field Model, identify three positives for returning to school now and three negatives for going back to school now.

Three positives for going back to school now: You can take advantage of the increased tuition benefits from the hospital. You begin working on the next phase of your career now instead of waiting until the children are all in school. You may be able to work out a more flexible schedule to enable you to go back to school.

Three negatives for returning to school now: It will be difficult to arrange a schedule that takes into account your rotations and your husband's schedule. The children are young and are still very needy of your time. Money is an issue; although the tuition benefits are generous, there will still be out-of-pocket expenses.

3. Are there any alternative solutions to this situation?

Raising a young family is a challenge regardless of the parents' work schedules, but to attempt to coordinate two difficult schedules and depend on babysitters to fill the gaps can appear almost overwhelming. Adding to the situation a full-time wage earner who may not have enough "free" time to attend on-site classes and complete homework only contributes to a difficult—but not impossible—school situation.

Instead of returning to school full-time, is there a possibility of returning to school on a part-time basis? Do any of the colleges offer weekend programs? With all the new technology available for learning, perhaps a look into distance-learning programs, whether video conferencing or computer-based classes, is worthwhile. Distance-learning programs do not require attendance as often as the more traditional classroom courses, and they enable adult learners to study when it is more convenient for them—even in the middle of the night. Given all the restrictions of your situation, distance-learning opportunities, at least for a portion of the degree, may be worth considering.

Another option is to speak with the nurse manager to see if your work schedule can be arranged to accommodate a school schedule. Many managers, in support of their employees returning to school, often will at least attempt a schedule change to accommodate both work and school. Perhaps this would be a good time to offer to work permanent nights or weekends or even take a Baylor position.

4. What would be an implementation schedule for the desired change?

It is said that there is no better time than right now to begin, so in keeping with that thought, you have decided that a distance program on a part-time basis for the first year is the best alternative at this point. By going part-time, you can still devote a fair amount of time to your growing family, yet you have not put off the decision to return to school. In reviewing your option to at least begin some course work on-line, you have kept in mind some of the issues about needing to be more available for your family and to be able to schedule coursework around your work schedule.

Once all the alternatives have been reviewed and one has been chosen, it is imperative to set up a timeline. Unless you are sure what school you would like to attend, at least one semester is needed for research and application. It is better to spend the time upfront assessing all the potential alternatives than to complete two or three classes only to find that the rest of the program does not meet your expectations.

Case Scenario 16-2

Regardless of where one works, change is a constant factor and, in most situations, inevitable. Identify one issue in the workplace that you feel needs to be changed in some manner. For example, a process may be in place that can be revised or dramatically improved, such as the procedure to check the unit code carts to ensure daily compliance. Another example of a needed change is to improve reports between shifts.

In this exercise, a priority issue that can be changed through the positive action of a nurse leader is identified to improve client, staff, or system health or behavior. Situational determinants and those influencing factors surrounding the identified problem or situation are assessed. Alternative strategies for change are devised, keeping in mind the diverse needs, priorities, and requirements of the system and organization.

Case Considerations

1. After discussion with a nurse leader, select an issue that requires change because of a perceived or an actual conflict.
2. Analyze and research issues surrounding the problem. Look for alternative solutions in the literature and among "experts."
3. Determine at least three strategies for change as well as the positive and negative forces on each strategy.

4. Discuss the proposed implementation of the planned change.
5. Establish the criteria on which the planned change is evaluated.

Case Analysis

Many opportunities exist in the workplace for increasing efficiency and effectiveness while improving processes. Change often causes, either directly or indirectly, fears and stress among those who are affected. Change planned by those who will be the most affected has the most potential for acceptance. Organizational changes should not be a surprise to those who work in the environment, and if this type of change occurs frequently rather than occasionally, it can lead to dissatisfaction and distrust.

When a planned change is to occur, it is often helpful to ask the advice of those who have already experienced a similar change process. A literature review also is often a useful starting point for a change project, particularly if the change agent is not familiar with a similar circumstance. Once the relevant information about the proposed situation is known, alternative solutions to solving the issue can be devised, with positives and negatives delineated for each alternative. Usually, the alternative with the fewest negatives is the one to consider most strongly for implementation. An implementation schedule is then developed, along with criteria that will measure the success of the project once completed.

■ KEY POINTS

1. Change is never easy, especially when many different types of people are concerned in a diverse health care environment.
2. Change can be more accepted if those who are the most likely to be affected by the results of the change have input into some of the decisions regarding the proposed changes.
3. Applying the work of a traditional theorist to the change process is a great way to outline the steps that are needed for a successful implementation. Lewin's Force Field Model is one that applies easily, enabling focused work on the benefits and disadvantages of different alternative solutions. Other theorists to consider in this change project include Lippitt et al. (1958), Havelock (1973), and Rogers (1983).
4. Regardless of the theory used, the change process has the following among its core concepts: assessment, planning, implementation of the change strategy, evaluation of the change, and stabilization of the change.

5. A change agent should be chosen early in the process to be the responsible person for ensuring that the change actually occurs.
6. Expect a variety of responses to the change process and the resulting scenario. No one responds in the same manner, but the most common response to change is resistance.

Case Scenario 16-3

You are team leader on the night shift, which includes two permanent certified nurses aides (CNAs) who have worked the floor for more than 20 years. They provide moderately good care when asked, but they are not exactly self-starters who look for opportunities to keep themselves busy. A new nursing graduate, Michael, started on the night shift a month ago. Michael used to work as a CNA on the floor while he was going through nursing school, and he had great rapport with the other two CNAs. Now, however, they barely speak to him, only grudgingly assist him when asked, and often don't even complete assignments that he asks them to do. In fact, they are doing only the minimal work for all the registered nurses on the floor and are frequently found talking together at the nurses' station. Michael, on the other hand, is certainly a team player who provides excellent nursing care and works well with everyone else on the floor.

As the team leader, you don't want to lose any of the permanent night-shift staff over this conflict; however, other staff tell you that the workplace is becoming increasingly uncomfortable. Michael has not yet mentioned anything directly to you, but you have heard that he was in the Human Resources Department inquiring about transfer policies.

Case Considerations

1. As the team leader on the night shift, what are your responsibilities to the staff in this situation?
2. Identify the conflict in this scenario.
3. Is gender an issue in this scenario? Discuss whether gender is ever an issue in nursing.
4. What are some of the obvious causes of the conflict situation?
5. Discuss some of the more obscure reasons that may be contributing to this conflict situation.
6. Is this a conflict on the intrapersonal, interpersonal, or organizational level, and why?

7. Describe some of the conflict resolution techniques that you, as team leader, can implement in this situation.
8. Describe at least two conflict resolution techniques that could be suggested to Michael.
9. What is the responsibility of the rest of the staff in this situation to both Michael and the two CNAs?
10. As team leader, what are some of your alternatives for solving this issue? Which one will you choose, and why?

Case Analysis

Conflict in the workplace, especially interpersonal conflict resulting from different personalities and expectations, is quite common. The one complicating factor in this particular scenario is that Michael was once in the same position as the two CNAs he now supervises, which results in conflict and an uneasy work situation. Regardless of the current situation, all parties must somehow learn to work together to provide good patient care delivery on the floor. Leadership must take an active part in resolving this conflict by encouraging and demonstrating open communication among all the participants.

■ KEY POINTS

1. Conflict is a component of change, but not all change brings conflict.
2. There are three main types of conflict: intrapersonal, interpersonal, and organizational. Sometimes, a conflict situation may manifest in all three types.
3. Leadership on the unit needs to intervene in this scenario before personnel are lost and the level of patient care declines.
4. Open communication is a key component in any successful conflict resolution situation.

References

Bennis, W., Benne, K., & Chinn, R. (1969). *The planning of change* (2nd ed.). New York: Holt, Rinehart, and Winston.

Filley, A. C. (1975). *Interpersonal conflict resolution.* Glenview, IL: Scott, Foresman.

Havelock, R. G. (1973). *The change agent's guide to innovation in education.* Englewood Cliffs, NJ: Educational Technology.

Lewin, K. (1951). *Field theory in social science.* New York: Harper & Row.

Lippit, R., Watson, J., & Westley, B. (1958). *The dynamics of planned change.* New York: Harcourt, Brace.

Rogers, E. M. (1983). *Diffusion of innovations* (3rd ed.). New York: Free Press.

Senge, P. M. (1990). *The fifth discipline: The art and practice of leading organizations.* New York: Doubleday.

Suggested Readings

Bass, B. (1980). *Bass and Stodgill's handbook of leadership.* New York: Free Press.

Bennis, W. (1989). *On becoming a leader.* Reading, MA: Addison-Wesley.

Bennis, W., & Nannus, B. (1985). *Leaders: The strategies for taking charge.* New York: Harper & Row.

Burns, J. M. (1978). *Leadership.* New York: Harper & Row.

Covey, S. (2000). *Change agents: New rules for communicating with employees.* Salt Lake City, UT: Franklin Covey.

Daft., R. L., & Marcic, D. (2001). *Understanding management* (3rd ed.). Philadelphia: Harcourt College.

Duck, J. D. (1993, November/December). Managing change: The art of balancing. *Harvard Business Review,* 109–118.

Fielder, F. (1967). *A theory of leadership effectiveness.* New York: McGraw-Hill.

Forni, P. M. (2002). *Choosing civility: The twenty-five rules of considerate conduct.* New York: St. Martin's Press.

Forte, P. S. (1997). The high cost of conflict. *Nursing Economic$, 15* (3), 119–123.

Gantz, N. R. (2002). The preservation of core values during times of chaos and conflict. *Pediatric Intensive Care Nursing, 3* (1), 9–12.

Greenfield, L. J. (1999). Doctors and nurses: A troubled partnership. *Annals of Surgery, 230,* 279–288.

Griggith, J. (1999). *The well-managed health care organization.* Chicago: Health Administration Press.

Gross, J. J. (2002) Emotion regulation: Affective, cognitive, and social consequences. *Psychophysiology, 39* (3), 281–291.

Henry, J. (2003). Positive organizations. *Psychologist, 16* (3), 138–139.

Henry, L. G., & Henry, J. D. (1999). *Reclaiming soul in health care.* Chicago: American Hospital Association.

Hersey, P., & Blanchard, K. (2000). *Management of organizational behavior* (8th ed.). Englewood Cliffs, NJ: Prentice Hall.

Herzberg, F. (1968, January/February). One more time: How do you motivate employees? *Harvard Business Review,* 53–62.

Iacono, M. (2003). Conflict, communication and collaboration: Improving relationships between nurses and physicians. *Journal of PeriAnesthesia Nursing, 18* (1), 42–46.

Ingersoll, G. L., Kirsch, J. C., Merk, S. E., & Lightfoot, J. (2000). Relationship of organizational culture and readiness for change to employee commitment to the organization. *Journal of Nursing Administration, 30* (1), 11–20.

Jones, T. S., & Bodtker, A. (2001) Mediating with heart in mind: Addressing emotion in mediation practice. *Negotiation Journal, 17* (3), 217–244.

Kotter, J. (1990). What leaders really do. *Harvard Business Review, 68,* 104.

Marquis, B. L., & Huston, C. J. (2000). *Leadership roles and management functions* (3rd ed.). Philadelphia: J. B. Lippincott.

Pillutla, M. M., & Murnighan, J. K. (1997) Unfairness, anger, and spite: Emotional rejections of ultimatum offers. *Organizational Behavior and Human Decision Processes, 68* (3), 208–224.

Rowland, H. S., & Rowland, B. L. (1997). *Nursing administration handbook* (4th ed.). Gaithersburg, MD: Aspen Publishers.

Shapiro, D. L. (2002). Negotiating emotions. *Conflict Resolution Quarterly, 20* (1), 67–82.

Umiker, W. (1997). Collaborative conflict resolution. *Health Care Supervisor, 15* (3), 70–75.

Wolper, L. (1999). *Health care administration planning, implementing and managing organized delivery systems* (3rd ed.). Gaithersburg, MD: Aspen Publishers.

Yukl, G. (1998). *Leadership in organizations* (4th ed.). Upper Saddle River, NJ: Prentice Hall.

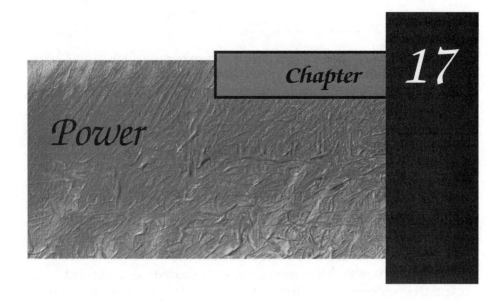

Chapter 17

Power

Essential Concepts of Power

Effective leaders are aware of the use and misuse of power and of its effects on those they work with in the health care setting. Nurses have tremendous potential for applying their power, yet for a variety of reasons, few successfully apply this skill to the workplace. People in management and leadership positions often display various degrees of power by virtue of the position they hold. One can also show power because of special expertise about a certain topic, because of the people they know, or even because of the clothes that they wear and the way in which they carry themselves. The simple act of decision-making is a demonstration of power—and an action that a registered nurse does frequently throughout the day.

Defining Power

- Power is the generalized capacity or potential of an individual that enables that person to get others to do something they would not ordinarily do.

- Power involves a relationship between two people. One cannot have power in isolation.
- Power is the ability to influence others to change their behavior or their thinking.

Levels of Power

- Personal power is closely related to how comfortable that person is with his or her perception of power and how others are influenced to change their thinking or actions.
- Experts are often viewed as having more power than those without that expertise, and they may be looked on as being more effective than those with a lesser perceived power base.
- Professional power arises from a person's credentials and what expertise is identified to others, both inside and outside the health care setting.
- Some in an organization are always viewed internally as being more powerful than others. Perhaps these people are perceived as being more powerful because of organizational affiliations, the committees they represent, or the specialty in which they work. Many times, decisions are affected by those with alleged organizational power rather by those with extensive knowledge.
- Nursing often has the organizational and professional power base to influence critical health care decisions. What is sometimes lacking, however, is the perceived personal power and beliefs in success.

Sources of Power

- Expert power is derived from a person having special knowledge or skills that others need or want. For example, a clinical nurse specialist in critical care is sought out by critical care staff for her expertise in balloon pumping techniques when a patient has difficulty maintaining a blood pressure on the pump.
- Legitimate power is also known as positional power. It is derived from where one's place is on the organizational chart, and depending on that placement, it is how much power one can demand or expect from others. Legitimacy also delineates the nurse's degree of authority. Just because someone has knowledge and a leadership position within the organization does not always mean that they are sought after for their opinions.
- Referent power, which is also known as charismatic power, is more personal than the other types of power. Nurses with significant referent power have a strong influence over others. Trust and respect are hallmarks of a referent power base, as is instilling confidence in followers.

- Reward power and coercive power are used to either reward or punish others, respectively, with fear being a common emotion (but especially in coercive power) if someone does not meet expectations. An example of reward power is the manager's ability to grant an additional weekend off if the staff nurse works two Friday nights in a row, whereas a manager applying coercive power would threaten to have the staff nurse work three weekends in a row if she calls off with one more sick day, regardless of the staff nurse's rationale.
- Connection power can be summed up as "it's not what you know, but who you know." Not everyone in a leadership position has a power base, and many times, even a secretary has a significant amount of power.
- Knowledge is power, and many use information power to their advantage. When the emergency room requests a medical-surgical bed, a charge nurse has information power when he or she knows that a patient is being actively discharged during the phone call but states that no beds are available.

Empowerment

- Empowerment is facilitating participation by others in the decision-making process, resulting in equal distribution of power between the manager and staff.
- The astute nurse manager will provide leadership opportunities for the staff members so that they feel empowered and want to assist in problem-solving for the unit.
- Understanding and being able to apply the basic concepts of power enables beginning nurses to be more effective in their decisions, both for themselves and for their patients.
- To secure nursing's future as a significant voice in American politics, individual nurses need to demonstrate their power, whether through voting for the right candidate, writing to legislators, or lobbying for a health care-related cause.

CASE SCENARIOS

Guided Case Scenario 17-1

Chris is the manager of the telemetry unit. On this particular unit, a problem exists with the staff and their poor morale. The moral issue has a variety of reasons, including a very busy work-load, demanding physicians who are not as collegial as they could be, and a high turnover rate of new people who leave within a year. Almost half of the staff has been employed on the telemetry unit for more than 10 years. The new people who are leaving are not necessarily new to nursing, however, because a registered nurse must have a minimum of 1 year of experience to apply for a position on the unit.

When Chris asked those who resigned why they decided to leave, many of them said that they felt powerless in their daily work. Many of the senior staff members concur. One of Chris' goals for the new year is to enhance the staff's personal level of empowerment.

Case Considerations

1. What are some of the sources of power found on Chris' unit, and what types of power are they?
2. Identify several issues adding to the feeling of powerlessness among the staff who are leaving
3. Would there be any feelings of powerlessness among those staff who are not leaving, and why?
4. How would Chris begin to empower his subordinates?
5. Describe some of the techniques that Chris could suggest to his staff not only to empower them but also to encourage power building within the institution.

Case Analysis

1. What are some of the sources of power found on Chris' unit, and what types of power are they?

   One of the most complicated functions of a manager in daily operations is dealing with the many personalities and abilities of staff members. Two significant issues behind the low morale on this unit may be the relationship between the physicians and nurses and the high turnover rate of newly employed personnel.

   With half the staff having more than 10 years of experience on the telemetry floor, a great deal of expert power is available among these nurses who have attained a certain level of knowledge. When compared to the newer nurses, these experienced nurses also hold legitimate power, which is derived from the position of tenure that these nurses hold on the unit. With connection power, it is not necessarily what you know,

and many of these long-term nurses have forged work relationships with the physicians that the newer nurses have not
had time to develop. There may even be evidence of reward or
coercive power being used in this setting by the senior nurses
toward the junior nurses.

Regardless of the time of tenure, any of the nurses may hold
referent or charismatic power, resulting in many who want to
be associated with these nurses simply because of their high
levels of trust and respect. Information power is another type
of power that does not depend on tenure or on personal relationships to be effective; this type of power comes simply from
having a certain knowledge base that others desire.

2. Identify several issues adding to the feeling of powerlessness
   among the staff who are leaving.

   Chris needs to dig a little deeper as to why his staff feels so
   powerless before any assumptions are made and solutions are
   suggested. At first glance, several issues come to mind about
   the source of staff powerlessness. Some of these issues include
   a significant number of the staff having been there for more
   than 10 years, demanding physicians, a heavy workload, and
   constantly changing coworkers.

3. Would there be any feelings of powerlessness among those
   staff who are not leaving, and why?

   The scenario suggests that not only are the newer nurses
   leaving but that the more senior ones are just as unhappy and
   have feelings of powerlessness. These feelings of powerlessness, however, may be different from those among the personnel who are leaving. It is difficult to work in an environment
   with constantly changing personnel. Training new nurses and
   staff requires a certain investment of time and trust, and when
   these staff leave after a short period, it can result in frustration
   for the remaining staff and a higher workload being already
   added to a stressful day.

   Although the more tenured nurses have worked with the
   current physicians for years, this does not mean that they do
   not wish for a more collegial work relationship. Challenging
   physicians who treat nurses as subordinates rather than team
   members can easily become another stressor, especially when
   communication is lacking and expectations are mixed. Added
   to the stress of an already busy environment and a high staff

turnover, this situation can cause even experienced nurses to feel disempowered.

4. How would Chris begin to empower his subordinates?

To empower his subordinates, Chris needs to share some of his power with others. By sharing this power, Chris is enabling his staff to partake in the decision-making process by sharing information and holding them accountable for the results. Creativity and risk taking are expected, encouraging personal and professional growth.

One can do several things to empower others. One of the most important is to delegate an assignment that historically the leader has completed. All the necessary information and known expectations should also be provided so that the delegate can have a successful experience. Much satisfaction can be gained from doing a task that was previously someone else's responsibility, doing that task well, and receiving positive recognition. One point to make when empowering someone is to ensure that the delegator does not relinquish the requisite power, authority, and accountability for the task.

Employees who are empowered either have the skills to be successful or are given opportunities to learn the skills needed to complete the assignments. It would be contradictory to expect someone to take on an assignment if they do not have the knowledge, so part of Chris's responsibility as manager is to ensure that his staff has the necessary training. In addition, any departmental barriers should be decreased—or even eliminated—to facilitate the staff's empowerment. It is difficult to change a situation through empowerment if all the time is spent dealing with organizational issues.

Chris also needs to understand that not everyone wants to feel empowered. There will always be nurses who do not want to take on additional responsibilities and accountability for unit functioning. Finally, Chris needs to do a personal inventory of his own skill set and, in his role of resolving conflicts, act as a mentor, both motivating and fostering collegiality among coworkers.

5. Describe some of the techniques that Chris could suggest to his staff not only to empower them but also to encourage power building within the institution.

Chris not only can make empowering opportunities happen on the telemetry floor but also can encourage his staff to develop their own sense of empowerment. Several things one can do to appear more powerful: (1) appearing powerful to others through dress, demeanor, actions, and communications; (2) understanding the organization's priorities, and making yourself available to assist the organization in reaching its goals through committee work, communications, or any other needed method; (3) joining committees that will increase one's visibility in the organization; (4) taking on tasks and responsibilities that will potentially result in specific people becoming aware of the outcomes; (5) developing new skills, and strengthening others; and (6) learning to empower others, because it is through others that work is accomplished.

Case Scenario 17-2

A new nurse, Sandy, is scheduled to begin orientation on the unit next week, and you are the designated preceptor. Sandy did her 200-hour leadership clinical rotation on the unit, and it was because of the nursing staff that she decided to apply for the open position. Her clinical evaluations by the staff were excellent; however, several said that she needed to be more assertive in dealing with coworkers, patients, and physicians. The experienced nurses who evaluated Sandy sensed that she was unsure of her decisions and, at times, almost appeared timid, yet they were unanimous in saying that she should be hired.

Case Considerations

1. Is there a need for Sandy to become more assertive if she is already clinically competent for a new registered nurse?
2. How do you develop an orientation plan that includes acquiring a sense of personal empowerment?
3. Discuss some key areas on which you will focus in helping Sandy to become more empowered.
4. What is the responsibility of the staff in Sandy's orientation? Of others in the organization?
5. Are there some issues that you may want to pay less attention to in the orientation process?
6. Who else will you involve in Sandy's orientation, and why?

Case Analysis

Being a new graduate nurse is not easy for anyone, regardless of the setting. Sandy has an advantage, though, in taking a position on the unit where she completed her preceptorship. She should at least be somewhat familiar with the daily routine, the types of patients the unit receives, some of the physicians and their specific orders, and most importantly, with staff that she worked with as a student. For someone who has a reserved personality, familiarity is important and can make them feel more comfortable and at ease.

As a preceptor, one of the things that you can do early on is to ensure that Sandy has a comfort level with those issues that she will encounter on a daily basis. To assist Sandy in becoming more self-powerful is to let her achieve successes early on, partly to build her confidence and partly to let others see that she is competent.

■ KEY POINTS

1. A new person needs to understand early on which issues are important to resolve within the organization. Every organization has certain beliefs about power and authority, such as who is powerful and who has authority decisions.
2. A preceptor can make or break an orientee's experience in the hospital, leading to whether the orientee is interested not only in remaining on the unit but also in staying employed in the organization.
3. A person who has a timid personality can also be seen as powerful in certain situations. It just takes the right situation.
4. Everyone on the unit has the responsibility to assist a new graduate in becoming successful, and that includes participating in or creating situations in which a new graduate can build early, visible achievements.
5. Clinical competency should not be an immediate expectation of a new graduate nurse; instead, safe care should be the goal.

Suggested Readings

Bass, B. (1980). *Bass and Stodgill's handbook of leadership*. New York: Free Press.
Bennis, W. (1989). *On becoming a leader*. Reading, MA: Addison-Wesley.
Bennis, W., & Nannus, B. (1985). *Leaders: The strategies for taking charge*. New York: Harper & Row.
Bower, F. L. (2000). *Nurses taking the lead: Personal qualities of effective leadership*. Philadelphia: W. B. Saunders.
Burns, J. M. (1978). *Leadership*. New York: Harper & Row.

Cummings, S. H. (1995). Attila the Hun versus Attila the Hen: Gender social-ization of the American nurse. *Nursing Administrative Quarterly, 19* (2), 19–29.

Daft., R. L., & Marcic, D. (2001). *Understanding management* (3rd ed.). Philadel-phia: Harcourt College.

Fielder, F. (1967). *A theory of leadership effectiveness.* New York: McGraw-Hill.

Fitzpatrick, J. J. (1997). The power of politics and partnerships. *Applied Nursing Research, 10* (4), 167.

Griggith, J. (1999). *The well-managed health care organization.* Chicago: Health Administration Press.

Hersey, P., & Blanchard, K. (2000). *Management of organizational behavior* (8th ed.). Englewood Cliffs, NJ: Prentice Hall.

Laschinger, H. K., & Wong, C. (1999). Staff nurse empowerment and collective accountability: Effect on perceived productivity and self-rated work effec-tiveness. *Nursing Economic$, 17* (6), 308–316.

Marquis, B. L., & Huston, C. J. (2000). *Leadership roles and management functions* (3rd ed.). Philadelphia: J. B. Lippincott.

Rodwell, C. M. (1996). An analysis of the concept of empowerment. *Journal of Advanced Nursing, 23,* 305–315.

Rowland, H. S., & Rowland, B. L. (1997). *Nursing administration handbook* (4th ed.). Gaithersburg, MD: Aspen Publishers.

Tebbitt, B. V. (1993). Demystifying organizational empowerment. *Journal of Nursing Administration, 23* (1), 18–23.

Wolper, L. (1999). *Health care administration planning, implementing and managing organized delivery systems* (3rd ed.). Gaithersburg, MD: Aspen Publishers.

Yukl, G. (1998). *Leadership in organizations* (4th ed.). Upper Saddle River, NJ: Prentice Hall.

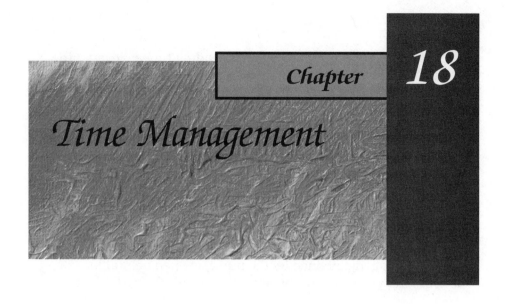

Chapter 18

Time Management

Essential Concepts of Time Management

One of the primary issues with nurses today is the lack of time to spend at the bedsides of their patients. Yet, if one looks at all the time that is wasted because of incorrectly delegated tasks, poor decision-making, and unavailability of equipment and supplies, it is easy to understand the need for improved time management skills. Many people, including patients, their families, physicians, allied health professionals, and coworkers, place demands on a registered nurse (RN), so it should be no surprise that the shift usually ends before everything is completed.

General Time Management Issues

- Several different methods exist to assist in developing time management skills. The first and most critical step is to decide on the final result. What is it that you hope to accomplish? By when? Are there any constraints?
- The Pareto Principle (Koch, 1999) states that only 20% of our efforts ends in 80% of the resulting consequences, so we need to focus on

what is really important rather than spending time on every little detail. Nurses, unfortunately, spend a great deal of wasted time searching for those things that are necessary for patient care, such as intravenous pumps, missing medications, and a missed meal, or waiting for a physician to call back with a needed order.

- To use time effectively, the nurse needs to understand approximately how much time a project or a task will take to complete. Many nurses spend less time on direct patient care than they may perceive—generally around a third of their total time. Charting, reporting, admission, and discharge procedures as well as performing care and tasks that could potentially be delegated round out the nurse's day.
- An activity log, maintained by the nurse, is often helpful in determining where time may be wasted or misdirected.

Strategies of Time Management

- When a significant amount of work needs to be done, it often helps to clarify the end result, because this helps to put smaller issues into perspective. Expectations of all shift team members are identified, including what tasks and outcomes are necessary for optimal patient care.
- The desired outcomes, or the expected results, need to be clear and communicated to all who work with a specific patient population. Once the outcomes are known and understood, the team can work effectively and efficiently toward those goals.
- Items are prioritized in the order that they need to be accomplished and by the expertise required. First-level priorities are the life-threatening (or potentially life-threatening) situations that place patients, staff, or families at risk. Second-level priorities are those activities that are essential to safety. Third-level priorities are those activities that are necessary to carry out patient care.

Application of Time Management Strategies

- After the crucial step of prioritizing, several additional techniques can be applied to maximize the manager's time. To plan appropriately, a correct estimate of the time needed to complete an activity must be made so that the more important activities are completed first. Planning for the manager is necessary, because certain daily functions, such as reviewing the staffing pattern, need to occur without fail.
- It is extremely helpful to have the necessary items available when they are needed so that one does not have to "hunt" for missing or

misplaced objects. When the environment is supportive, more time can be spent on direct patient care.

- Shift reports can organize a shift right at the beginning, so extra care should be placed on ensuring that the needed information is given on eliminating old or nonessential data.
- A shift action plan is a written plan that delineates and prioritizes what care needs to be completed by the end of the shift and by whom. These plans should also include the times at which interventions should be completed.
- Patient roundings are most effective at the beginning and at the completion of a shift. Rounds help the nurse in assessing both the patient and the room. Does that patient appear as the report stated? Are the IVs labeled and in need of a change? Is the room stocked? Managers should be rounding on all the patients for a variety of reasons.
- At the completion of the shift, the desired outcomes that were set at the beginning of the shift should be reviewed for completion.

Strategies to Increase Personal Productivity

- One way to increase personal productivity is to change your sleep patterns slightly, by getting up 1 hour earlier in the morning or by staying up 1 hour later in the evening.
- A useful strategy to incorporate into a busy life is to take advantage of "downtimes" and use them for those activities that require quiet time. Also, by decreasing unwanted distractions, one can add minutes or, perhaps, even hours of productivity to the day by not answering the phone or talking to casual visitors.

CASE SCENARIOS

Guided Case Scenario 18-1

More than 6 months ago, you graduated from a BSN program and started a permanent night position at the local hospital. Working as an RN has been a goal of yours for the last 10 years, while you worked as a phlebotomist to support your growing family. Although you work 5 days a week, between your professional life, your home life, and your volunteer work, you feel like you are never caught up. In fact, you cannot say no when someone asks you to do overtime, which is at least 12 additional hours a week.

You thought that doing this extra time at work would help you to become more organized; however, you are still as disorganized as when you began your new job. In fact, you are late every day in trying to complete your reports and to make sure that everything that needs to be done is completed.

One of the goals that you have set for yourself—and your spouse wholeheartedly agrees—is that you begin work on your graduate degree as soon as possible. You mailed your application to the university last week. You want to begin course work, but you are feeling so overwhelmed with everything that you are seriously reconsidering your application.

Case Considerations

1. Identify some time management issues of the new graduate nurse in this scenario.
2. List, in descending order, the time management priorities for this nurse and why they are in that particular order.
3. What are some strategies that would help this nurse to plan an effective use of time at work?
4. Discuss some strategies that may assist this nurse with time management skills for personal time.

Case Analysis

1. Identify some time management issues of the new graduate nurse in this scenario.

So many time management issues surround this new graduate that it is hard to decide which is the most demanding. The easiest way to identify the time management issues in this case is to break them down into professional/work, professional/career, and personal.

Working 40 hours a week is not enough for this new nurse; another 12 hours of overtime are added weekly because he cannot say "no." The workday is disorganized, which becomes more evident as the daily overtime continues. Time management issues in the professional/career category are simple: This new nurse does not have adequate time for all his current obligations, including family and volunteer work, and he wants to add another huge commitment—graduate school.

Finally, the concerns surrounding his personal life affect both of the professional spheres. The main issue here is the amount of time not spent with the family. Obligations to volunteer work can augment family and personal life, or they can add to the burden of attempting to manage multiple commitments.

2. List, in descending order, the time management priorities for this nurse and why they are in that particular order.

   Everyone has different priorities in his or her life, with some placing home life over work and some placing their professional career over family. One of the most important notions to remember when looking at a busy life is that everything has to be in balance. When one's work life is out of balance, it will affect the stability of one's personal life, and vice versa.

   This nurse clearly needs to reflect on what is the most important issue at hand. Is it getting a handle on some of the disorganization of his daily work life? Is it a need to spend more time with his growing family? Is it returning to school to earn a graduate degree? Regardless of which becomes the priority, it will reflect upon the other areas. Time management techniques can be easily applied to both work situations and one's personal life, because the goals are the same: effective use of limited time and resources.

3. What are some strategies that would help this nurse to plan an effective use of time at work?

   The first thing this nurse needs to do when planning an effective use of time at work is to reflect on the actual use of time, on what activities are being completed, and on what activities are being left undone because of lack of time. What percentage of time is being spent on direct patient care? What percentage of time is being spent on charting and reporting? What percentage of time is being spent on admission and discharge procedures? What percentage of time is being spent on professional communication? Moreover, what percentage of time is being spent on activities that could be effectively delegated to someone else? When the nurse has a better sense of time usage, he can better plan how to rearrange the work day. Is a lot of time being wasted because of searching for equipment and supplies that are not easily available? If so, then maybe the real problem is not so much disorganization as a lack of needed supplies and something that, perhaps, the manager can better address.

   Many experienced nurses suggest keeping a daily log with memory joggers, much like students use during their clinicals to help them organize their days. The assigned patients could be listed in one column, with scheduled activities, such as medications, treatments, scheduled tests, labs, and so on, written across the top. This type of log will assist the nurse in seeing at a glance which patient needs what activity and when, and it can help when the RN is delegating certain patient care tasks and responsibilities to other team members. Other helpful tools that can assist the nurse in organizing time are shift reports and patient-focused rounds.

4. Discuss some strategies that may assist this nurse with time management skills for personal time.

Someone's personal life, like someone's work life, can also be a little disorganized, making the person feel like there is little time to complete tasks and enjoy life. A balance between work and home life needs to be achieved. Often, the pendulum swings in favor of a project coming due at work, then swings back in favor of family obligations at home.

What can be done to realize more free time in one's personal life? Like time management in the workplace, an inventory of daily events is helpful in assisting someone with understanding just where time is being spent. Is it watching TV? Talking on the phone? In traffic? Commuting? People are often unaware just how much time they spend in front of the TV or simply talking on the phone.

One way to simplify one's life is to control unwanted distractions, such as neighbors stopping in or taking phone calls that have little value. Paying bills once or twice a month and then immediately filing the paperwork is often helpful in controlling all the mail that continually clutters up the house. Use voice mail or an answering machine whenever possible to avoid lengthy phone calls that may be unwanted. Keeping the house as organized as possible gives a sense of having control over your environment and your life.

Case Scenario 18-2

You are the evening team leader for four staff members: one new RN graduate, one licensed practical nurse (LPN), and two nursing assistants. As a team, you have 22 patients. As you begin rounds, the following events are occurring: (1) Dr. Feelgood is waiting to discuss a medication error that was made 2 weeks ago, and he is being quite loud about the issue at the nursing station, where there are visitors; (2) the public toilet is overflowing, and waste is pouring

Table 18-1   Patients and Acuity Levels for Case Scenario 18-2

Patient Case Load	Patient Acuity Levels (4 = Highest)
Five are fresh postoperatives from the day shift, with IV medication needs at 4 and 6 hours plus intake and output	2, 2, 3, 3, and 4
You are expecting four more postoperatives, including two extensive bowel surgeries	2, 3, 3, and 4
Two will be discharged on tonight's shift and will need discharge teaching	1 and 1
Eight are medical, including six total care	1, 2, 3, 3, 3, 3, 4, and 4
One is critically ill and is waiting for a critical care bed, with four drips (two vasopressors) and vital signs every 15 minutes	4
Two are pscyhiatric (one bipolar and in the manic phase and one depressed)	2 and 3

out; (3) a visitor has fainted; and (4) the LPN on the team just broke off her engagement with her fiancé and is crying in a corner. Table 18-1 provides additional details regarding your patients and their acuity levels.

Case Considerations

1. Where does one even begin to plan for this shift?
2. What are the top three priorities for the shift, and why?
3. What are the three lowest priorities for the shift, and why?
4. Identify the activities that you will delegate and why are you delegating these activities.
5. Discuss your responsibility to the new RN graduate.
6. According to your state Board of Nursing, what are the delegation criteria that you need to keep in mind when delegating to unlicensed assistive personnel (UAPs)?

Case Analysis

Sometimes, it may appear that everything is a crisis and that every situation demands immediate attention, especially when few people are available to help. Remembering the Pareto Principle, what are the critical situations on which you can focus your effort to maximize the results? Which of the above situations can wait?

Which of the situations need immediate attention and cannot be delegated? An effective time manager considers the entire picture even before one decision is made to ensure that a priority item is, in fact, addressed.

■ KEY POINTS

1. Each state's Board of Nursing has delegation criteria for UAPs, and this criteria needs to be kept in mind for all delegation situations.
2. Likewise, the health care institution should have a policy in place that addresses what activities UAPs can do within their scope of practice.
3. It is easy to look at an entire scenario as a crisis, but to manage the situation effectively, the individual components need to be broken down into priorities. What needs to be addressed immediately or will have severe repercussions? What can be delayed until more assistance is rendered?
4. It is also easy to overwhelm a new graduate, so care must be taken to ensure an assignment that, while challenging, can be accomplished both effectively and safely by the end of the shift.
5. Team leaders often take on too much of the assigned tasks rather than delegating appropriately. As a team leader, you should ensure that the assignments you keep can be accomplished, knowing that you are responsible for the overall care provided by the entire team.
6. Sometimes, the loudest person demands immediate attention, and it just may be easier to address them sooner rather than later.

Reference

Koch, R. (1999). *The 80/20 principle: The secret to success by achieving more with less.* New York: Doubleday.

Suggested Readings

Burke, T. A., McKee, J. R., Wilson, H. C., Donahue, R. M., Batenhorst, A. S., & Pathak, D. S. (2000). A comparison of time-and-motion and self-reporting methods of work measurement. *Journal of Nursing Administration, 30* (3), 118–125.

Cardona, P., Tappen, R. M., Terrill, M., Acosta, M., & Eusebe, M. (1997). Nursing staff time allocation in long-term care. *Journal of Nursing Administration, 27* (2), 28–36.

Hansten, R. I., & Washburn, M. J. (1998). *Clinical delegation skills: A handbook for professional practice.* Aliso Viejo, CA: AACN.

Marquis, B. L., & Huston, C. J. (2000). *Leadership roles and management functions* (3rd ed.). Philadelphia: J. B. Lippincott.

Prescott, P. A., Ryan, J. W., & Thompson, K. O. (1991). Changing how nurses spend their time. *Image, 23* (1), 23–27.

Rowland, H. S., & Rowland, B. L. (1997). *Nursing administration handbook* (4th ed.). Gaithersburg, MD: Aspen Publishers.

Severance, J. S., & Cervantes, E. (1996).Time management training for home care workers. *Caring, 15* (5), 58–61.

Sullivan, E. J., & Decker, P. J. (2001). *Effective leadership and management in nursing* (5th ed.). Menlo Park, CA: Addison-Wesley.

Upenieks, V. B. (1998). Work sampling: Assessing nursing efficiency. *Nursing Management, 49* (4), 27–29.

UNIT

Evaluation

V

Chapter 19

Managing Outcomes

Essential Concepts of Outcome Management

A hallmark of a truly excellent health care facility is high quality standards not only for the care that is delivered but also for its positive outcomes. The development of total quality management (TQM) is generally attributed to W. Edward Deming and Joseph Juran, who both worked in the manufacturing industry during the 1950s. The concept of TQM, which is also known as quality improvement (QI), is to focus on the customer's needs while promoting a systematic process to continuously review, improve, and evaluate outcome measures. The focus on continuous QI differs from the older method of quality assurance, which emphasized inspecting results rather than focusing on the process of service delivery from the beginning to the end. Numerous methods and strategies are employed in the continuous QI process, but all center on the concept of improvement rather than being satisfied with the status quo.

Principles of Quality and Performance Improvement

- The early development of quality assurance in the health care industry focused on the maintenance and monitoring of minimum standards within a hospital system, with the goal being to identify errors predominantly in a retrospective review. The primary tool used to identify issues was the chart audit. The focus was on "what should have been done"—and was often punitive in nature—rather than on the best method to put in place so that the error was not repeated.

- TQM is also known as performance improvement, QI, and continuous QI. The concept of QI began with the work of Deming and Juran during the 1950s. It developed into a science that is a systematic, ongoing process to improve quality, and it is much more proactive in nature than the quality assurance process (Deming, 1986). The emphasis is on customer satisfaction and on "doing the right thing" to achieve customer confidence and, hopefully, repeat business.

- General principles of QI are multiple. However, key principles revolve around the structured system that encourages participation from all levels within the organization to improve identified processes.

- The focus in health care is on the customer. Each system has multiple customers, including patients and their families; health care providers, including nurses and physicians; insurance payers, regulatory agencies, and the community in which the organization exists.

- A key element in the QI process is that everyone, regardless of his or her position (e.g., Chief Executive Officer, employee in the laundry facility, or physician), is expected to participate. By encouraging, empowering, and trusting in their employees, organizations can initiate, implement, and maintain change more dramatically than those organizations that only place a certain level of employee in the QI process. This empowerment helps employees to understand that they have a stake in the success of the organization and are responsible for its success or failure. The goal of the individual process project determines who is invited to participate on the team, but those who are directly involved with the concern, along with a leader within the organization, often are included.

- The process of work delivery and its results, or outcomes, is the predominate focus of QI teams. Process is defined as a series of steps to produce an identified result. The goal is to improve the system, or all those factors that come together to achieve the desired outcome.

- A critical element to understand about the QI process is that it is a continuous, dynamic process that always presents an opportunity to improve.

Quality Improvement and Implications for Patient Care

- The primary thrust for engaging in a QI process is to improve patient care outcomes while decreasing costs. As a result of the QI process, patient care processes become more standardized, decreasing the costs of providing the care. The length of inpatient stays often decreases as well, because the care that is provided is more consistent with successful outcomes.

Improvement Strategies

- The Plan Do Check Act Cycle (Langley, Nolan, Norman, Provost, & Nolan, 1996) requires forward thinking and planning. The QI team must first decide what needs to be accomplished, then how one can identify what changes were made, and finally, did the change result in an improvement?
- FOCUS methodology applies the steps to the QI process, beginning with a Focus on the improvement opportunity, Organizing a team, Clarifying the process, Understanding the degree to which change is needed, and Selecting a solution for improvement (McLaughlin & Houston, 2003, p. 385).
- Both strategies work well with having flow diagrams applied. Flow diagrams are visuals that map out the steps in a given methodology.
- Benchmarking is the process of comparing one service or product against like services or products from outside the institution. Benchmarking identifies those with the lowest costs and the best outcomes, which result in the best practices. Benchmarking is a form of quality measurement, with the goal being to come as close as possible to the best practice, product, or process.
- Regulatory bodies, such as the Joint Commission on Accreditation of Healthcare Organizations (JCAHO; http://www.jcaho.org) and the National Council for Quality Assurance (http://www.ncqa.org) offer standards, information, and data to assist an agency's QI process.
- The balanced scorecard preidentifies four areas of critical importance to the organization, with all activities within the agency being measured against these standards. The idea is that for a process to be optimized, a balance must exist in the four areas.
- A storyboard is a method to illustrate the steps toward process achievement.

Data Application in the Quality Improvement Process

- A variety of charts are used to demonstrate the QI process.
- The time series chart illustrates the changes that occur in a process over time, allowing a team to track data points.

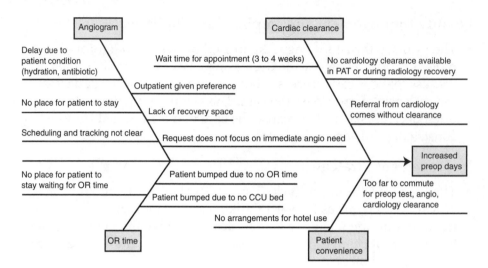

Figure 19-1   Root Cause/Fishbone Diagram.

- Additional charts to use in the QI process include the Pareto chart, the histogram, the flowchart, the fishbone diagram, pie charts, and check sheets (Figures 19-1 and 19-2). Data can be displayed in a variety of ways to get the necessary point across.

Quality Improvement and Risk Management

- Every organization requires a consistent methodology to enhance its success in achieving desirable patient outcomes. Application of the QI process has proven itself over time, in many different industries, and offers the best chance of successful outcomes for the patient, customers, and organization.
- The role of risk management in an organization is to prevent the loss of financial assets from injuries primarily to patients but also to employees, visitors, and medical staff. In the beginning, risk management focused on insurance and the transfer of risk dealing with lawsuits and malpractice issues, but today, it also includes the identification and prevention of situations that may be rectified before damages occur (Kongstvedt, 2002).
- The nurse manager has overall responsibility for quality initiatives in the patient care areas. The nurse manager always needs to be cognizant of any variances that occur outside of accepted patient care standards as well as any issues that place the organization at risk when families, employees, physicians, or community members are involved.

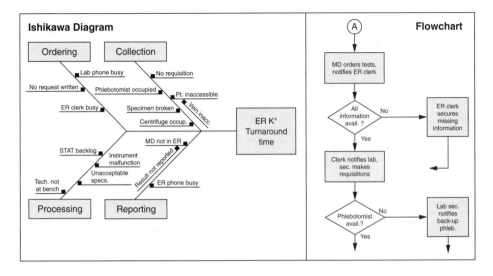

Check Sheet

Delays in production of Se K⁺ results from 1/1/91 to 1/7/91

Code/Delay Type		Mon	Tue	Wed	Thur	Fri	Sat	Sun	Total
A	Request not written by physician	I	I				I		3
B	Lab phone busy > 2 minutes	I		I		II		I	5
C	Phlebotomists unavailable	III	II	III	III	II	IIII	III	20
D	Requisition not ready	II	I	I	I	I	III	II	11
E	Patient inaccessible	I	I	II	I		II	I	8
F	Vein inaccessible	I		II		I	II		6
G	Centrifuge busy	II		I		I			4
H	Specimen broken	II		I				I	4
I	STAT backlog	III			I		II	I	7
J	Tech. not at bench	II		II		I	II	I	8
K	Unacceptable specimen	I	I		II		I	II	7
L	Lab. sec. unavailable to report	III		I		I	I		6
M	ER Phone not answered			I			II		3
N	MD not in ER	II		I		II		I	5
O	MD not answer page	I	I	II		II		II	8
P	Results not reported by ER sec.	II	I	II	I	III	II	II	13

Fiġure 19-2   Ishikawa Diagram, Flowchart, Check Sheet, Pareto Chart, and Control Chart. From *Clinical Laboratory Management Review,* November/December 1991, 5 (6), 448–462; © Clinical Laboratory Management Association, Inc.; all rights reserved. *(Figure continues on following page.)*

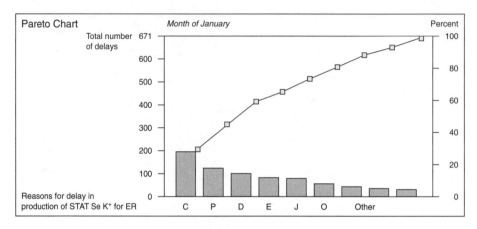

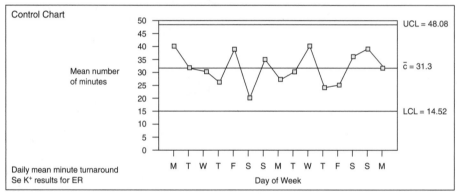

Figure 19-2   *(Continued.)*

CASE SCENARIOS

Guided Case Scenario 19-1

You are the team leader of a 50-bed surgical floor that receives a variety of patient diagnoses. One of the more problematic areas is the large intestinal surgeries, which run 4 to 5 days beyond the average length of stay in the United States and are complicated by high postoperative infection rates. When administrators ask the surgeons why their lengths of stays are so long, they say it is because the patients are more sick and less compliant with their postoperative care.

A multidisciplinary task force is forming to study the issue. You are asked to serve as cofacilitator. The committee is charged not only with making recommendations but also with implementing them and assisting in the evaluation of progress toward decreasing the length of stay and improving quality outcomes.

Case Considerations

1. Who should be invited to participate on the multidisciplinary committee, and why?
2. Identify the purpose and goals of the committee.
3. Discuss the process that the team could use in reviewing the quality indicators.
4. Describe several considerations regarding the extended length of stay for bowel surgeries at this facility.
5. What could the team suggest as ideas for improvement? What indicators will be used to measure progress toward meeting the goals?

Case Analysis

1. Who should be invited to participate on the multidisciplinary committee, and why?

One of the hallmarks of the continuous improvement process is to include members of various levels within the organization in the improvement procedure. If the primary quality problem deals more directly with physician and physician care, then it is prudent to have a physician champion as the other cofacilitator of the multidisciplinary committee.

Other key members of the committee could be a staff nurse who works on the surgical floor, a dietician, a social worker, representative key physicians, a case manager, and an administrator. Anyone from a discipline that is a stakeholder in improving outcomes could potentially become a member of this multidisciplinary committee.

2. Identify the purpose and goals of the committee.

The purpose of the committee is to improve the current length of stay and, optimally, patient outcomes for bowel surgeries through various methods. One goal of the committee is to reduce the average length of stay for a patient after bowel surgery to 5 days. Another goal could be to decrease the rate of postoperative infections from 15% to 6% within the first year of implementing the new protocols.

3. Discuss the process that the team could use in reviewing the quality indicators.

It is often helpful to have a change agent, who has no direct tie, coordinate the committee meetings and serve as a liaison between the committee and the administration. Committee members may be too close to some of the more controversial issues, and having someone who has no directly applicable stake in the outcome—other than wanting to have successful outcomes—temper the meeting is a good move. The change agent could communicate with the key administrator who is charged with decreasing the average length of stay and ensuring that the committee focuses on the parameters that need attention, not some obscure issues about which one particular committee member is concerned.

The meetings should be scheduled at a time when all committee members can attend, and then a schedule should be set several months, at minimum, in advance. The schedule should also be sent to the surgeons' offices so that there will be no confusion over scheduling operating room time during a meeting (unless an emergency occurs). Often, surgeons can be available midday, rather than first thing in the morning.

An agenda and any reading materials should be sent out at least a week ahead of time. Send these out too early, and they will get lost in the rest of the mail. Send these out too late, and they will not be read. An agenda helps everyone keep to task, and it makes follow-up and follow-through easier.

Quality indicators may be driven by the institution or the JCAHO. Either way, it is necessary to identify them early so that they can be tracked for compliance and improvement over time. In addition to length of stay, appropriate indicators may be cost per case and postoperative infection rates. With every meeting, the preidentified quality indicators should be discussed, tracked, and noted for improvement or decline.

4. Describe several considerations regarding the extended length of stay for bowel surgeries at this facility.

The physicians may feel that the patients are more sick than those at other area institutions, and they may be correct—or incorrect. It is easy to obtain comparative acuity data that looks at the same indicators at local, regional, and even nationally known institutions to discover whether clients at the hospital are, indeed, more sick or whether this is conjecture. One area to consider is the bowel preparation. Is it done at home, or are patients coming into the hospital and having it completed there, possibly adding an extra day or two to their length of stay? After surgery, how quickly is someone ambulating? When do the patients get to eat? Do they eat only after they have bowel sounds, or do they eat much sooner? What are the different nursing practices? Do many of the patients have similar comorbidities, and are they adding to the length of stay? What are the physician practices? A length of stay can be increased for many reasons, and a difference in physician practice is always a consideration.

5. What could the team suggest as ideas for improvement? What indicators will be used to indicate progress toward meeting the goals?

The first step in developing a QI plan is to identify potential indicators of quality, such as those described in the previous answer. The ultimate focus on choosing the indicators should be centered on patient care, with data driving the process change decisions. Quality indicators should also be linked to the organization's mission, goals, and vision, and they should be complementary rather than contrasting.

The easiest way to identify potential indicators of success toward meeting the committee's goal would be to reveal those indicators that directly affect decreasing length of stay for patients undergoing bowel surgery. Look at indicators such as admission and discharge dates, quality of care issues (e.g., infection rates), cost issues, functional status issues (e.g., ambulation), and finally, rates of patient satisfaction with not only the hospital stay but also the nursing and medical care. With any indicator, it is important to be able to measure in quantitative terms as much as possible so that consistent measures are obtained between evaluators.

Case Scenario 19-2

Data for your medical unit shows an increasing number of patients who are experiencing a postoperative site infection after undergoing bowel resections; this month alone, four such infections occurred. The unit manager just came from a meeting in which these data were presented by the Director of Case Management, the Director of Risk Management, the Infection Control Nurse, and the Vice President for Patient Care Services. The manager plans to take this information to the multidisciplinary task force but first wants concrete data to present. She turns to you and several other senior nurses to meet and identify some of the causative factors.

Case Considerations

1. How would you benchmark this information against other local and regional hospitals?
2. Describe the sentinel event review process and how an infection could develop into a sentinel event.
3. Develop a fishbone diagram for discovering the root cause of the increasing infection rate on the unit.
4. Using similar information, develop a flowchart, check sheet, Pareto chart, and control chart to discover the causative factors for the increasing infection rate on the unit.

Case Analysis

When attempting to unearth the causative factor for any patient care issue, it is crucial to remember that issues generally are multi-layered and not the result of a single cause. Performing a variety of explorations and displaying the data findings in different ways, such as a Pareto chart, a flowchart, and a fishbone diagram, often lead to discovery of the root cause of the patient care issue and can only augment the decision-making process.

■ KEY POINTS

1. Benchmarking is the method used to compare one institution's findings against those of other similar institutions.
2. When attempting to uncover the causes behind a result, it is important to keep in mind that it is generally a process, not a single factor, that contributes to the result.
3. A sentinel review is applied when a significant untoward event results in the death of or a serious injury to a patient.
4. Several different types of charts can be used to present data findings.
5. The time series chart enables the viewer to see the changes in quality over time.
6. The fishbone diagram, which is also known as the root cause diagram, allows visualization of the many causative factors that contribute to an issue.
7. A flowchart is an illustrated algorithm that attempts to define the cause-and-effect results of a problem.

8. By using the above-mentioned tools to discover the underlying factors of a problem, decision-making is made clearer for many issues.

References

Deming, W. E. (1986). *Out of the crisis*. Cambridge, MA: Center for Advanced Engineering Study.

Kongstvedt, P. (2002). *Managed care: What it is and how it works*. Gaithersburg, MD: Aspen Publishers.

Langley, G. J., Nolan, K. M., Norman, C. L., Provost, L. P., & Nolan, T. W. (1996). *The improvement guide*. San Francisco: Jossey-Bass.

McLaughlin, M., & Houston, K. (2003). Managing outcomes using an organizational improvement model. In P. Kelly-Heidenthal (Ed.), *Nursing leadership and management*. Clifton Park, NY: Delmar Learning.

Suggested Readings

Al-Assaf, A. F., & Schmele, J. (1997). *Total quality in health care*. Boca Raton, FL: St. Lucie Press.

Caldwell, C. (1998). *Handbook for managing change in healthcare*. Milwaukee, WI: ASQ Press.

Crosby, P. B. (1989). *Let's talk quality*. New York: McGraw-Hill.

Griffith, J. (1999). *The well-managed health care organization*. Chicago: Health Administration Press.

Grift, R. G., & Mosel, D. (1994). *Benchmarking in health care: A collaborative approach*. Chicago: American Hospital Publishing.

Institute of Medicine. (2001). *Crossing the quality chasm: A new health system for the 21st century*. Washington, D.C.: National Academy Press.

Joint Commission on Accreditation of Healthcare Organizations. (1998). *Comprehensive accreditation manual for hospitals*. Oakbrook, IL: Joint Commission on Accreditation of Healthcare Organizations.

King, K. M., & Teo, K. K. (2000). Integrating clinical quality improvement strategies with nursing research. *Western Journal of Nursing Research, 22* (5), 596–608.

Kitson, A. (2000). Toward evidence-based quality improvement: Perspectives from nursing practice. *International Journal of Quality in Health Care, 12* (6), 459–464.

Koivela, M., Paunonen, M., & Laippala, P. (1998). Prerequisites for quality improvement in nursing. *Journal of Nursing Management, 6* (6), 333–342.

Kongstvedt, P. (2001). *Essentials in managed care* (4th ed.). Gaithersburg, MD: Aspen Publishers.

Meisenheimer, C. G. (1997). *Improving quality.* Gaithersburg, MD: Aspen Publishers.

Rowland, H. S., & Rowland, B. L. (1997). *Nursing administration handbook* (4th ed.). Gaithersburg, MD: Aspen Publishers.

Shui, L., & Singh, D. A. (1998). *Delivering health care in America.* Gaithersburg, MD: Aspen Publishers.

Sultz, H. A., & Young, K. M. (1999). *Health care USA* (2nd ed.). Gaithersburg, MD: Aspen Publishers.

Wolper, L. (1999). *Health care administration planning, implementing and managing organized delivery systems* (3rd ed.). Gaithersburg, MD: Aspen Publishers.

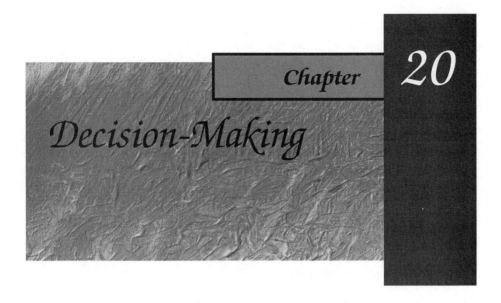

Chapter **20**

Decision-Making

Essential Concepts of Decision-Making

The hallmark of a successful and effective nurse leader is being able to take the components of problem-solving and critical thinking and use them to make decisions—and to make those decisions appropriately. Problem-solving focuses on analyzing a particular situation, with the result being that a decision is reached. Critical thinking is a broader activity, in which reasoning and creativity are applied in the process of arriving at a well-thought-out decision that takes into account alternative actions. The nursing process is a framework system of analysis that nurses can apply in making decisions, with the ability not only to assist the nurse in making decisions but to provide a mechanism for evaluating their decisions.

One instrument that may be helpful in making decisions is a decision-making grid. This tool helps to identify clearly the issues and the potential alternatives contained within a particular situation. Likewise, a Program Evaluation and Review Technique (PERT) is a flowchart that takes into account the decision timing and sequencing that are needed to complete a project. Other tools that can assist the nurse manager are decision trees and Gantt charts, which can be applied to most situations.

Application of the Critical Thinking Process

- Reflective thinking (Pesut & Herman, 1999) is a technique that is useful for revealing several sides of an issue and for evaluating a decision once it has been made.
- The problem-solving process involves six steps: identifying the issue, collecting data, developing alternative solutions to evaluate for appropriateness, selecting an alternative, implementing the selected alternative, and evaluating the effectiveness of the alternative.
- Critical thinking used the principles of both decision-making and the problem-solving process.

Management Tools Used in Decision-Making

- The decision-making grid outlines, in table format, different alternatives and the possible effects of a particular decision on the alternative.
- PERT assists the manager in timing issues with a chosen alternative by outlining the sequencing of events that must occur to complete the assignment (Finkler & Kovner, 2000).
- A decision tree is similar to a pro/con visual to assist the manager in making a decision. In a decision tree, different alternatives are delineated.
- A Gantt chart places the entire project on a timeline to facilitate its visualization.

Group Decision-Making

- Some decisions are best made by a group rather than by the manager alone.
- Advantages of group decision-making (Table 20-1) include ease of communication, promotion of cohesiveness, and greater likelihood of support for the change.
- Disadvantages of group decision-making (Table 20-1) include the potential for individual opinions to influence others, increased length of time for processing, and possible personal conflicts and disagreements.
- Several methods exist to facilitate group decision-making (Cawthorpe & Harris, 1999). In the nominal group technique, all opinions are valued, discussed, and voted upon. The Delphi group technique uses the same components as the nominal group technique, except that the group members do not meet face to face and, instead, use

Table 20-1   Advantages and Disadvantages of Groups

Advantages	Disadvantages
• Easy and inexpensive way to share information • Opportunities for face-to-face communication • Opportunity to become connected with a social unit • Promotion of cohesiveness and loyalty • Access to a larger resource base • Forum for constructive problem-solving • Support group • Facilitation of espirit de corps • Promotion of ownership of problems and solutions	• Individual opinions influenced by others • Individual identity obscured • Formal and informal role and status positions evolve—hierarchies • Dependency fostered • Time consuming • Inequity of time given to share individual information • Existence of nonfunctional roles • Personality conflicts

questionnaires to offer their responses. In the Delphi group technique, more people can participate, but it can take a longer time to come to a decision based on the number of participants and the breadth of the project.
- Consensus building is a technique that is used when all members of a group need to have buy-in to a decision. Consensus decision-making means that all members of the group can live with the final decision, not that they all agree to the decision in its entirety.
- Groupthink is the opposite of consensus building. In groupthink, all members of the group need to be in 100% agreement with the final decision. Members are not encouraged to offer their opinions freely, to disagree, and to debate. A manager needs to be aware of groupthink as a potential side effect of group decision-making.

Strategies to Effective Decision-Making

- Although many different strategies are available to help the nurse manager make effective decisions, it is always important to develop a good critical thinking process, asking as many questions as necessary to obtain complete information.
- Using a pro/con listing often helps you to clarify issues that affect a decision.
- Trusting your decision-making is crucial. Once a decision is made, stick with it, and do not second guess yourself.

CASE SCENARIOS

Guided Case Scenario 20-1

While making rounds at the beginning of your shift, you check in on Mr. Rodriguez, who has an insulin-dependent diabetes and was diagnosed at this hospital admission. Mr. Rodriguez' wife and two children (ages 8 and 10) are also in the room. He is sitting on his chair, with the new diabetic teaching kit in his lap, and looks mildly confused. He was admitted 4 days ago with complications caused by his disease, and you assumed that he had received all the appropriate and necessary diabetic teaching, including medication administration, to prepare him and his family for discharge. His English is nominal, his wife speaks only Spanish, but both children are bilingual. Your Spanish is nominal.

When you ask him about his comfort level and understanding of his disease, his children translate that he knows little and is actually quite nervous about the "shots." Apparently, someone did come in once to teach Mr. Rodriguez about diabetes, but that person never validated whether he understood or what he was able to understand. Mr. Rodriguez is scheduled to be discharged this morning. A patient in the Emergency Department is waiting for the bed.

Case Considerations

1. What is your immediate reaction to this situation?
2. After your initial reaction, describe your plan of action. Identify your priority. How does your critical thinking process guide your decision?
3. Identify others who may be able to assist in your decision-making.
4. Describe some of the factors that you considered while contemplating your alternative decisions.

Case Analysis

1. What is your immediate reaction to this situation?

A normal first reaction most likely would be that given the current situation, Mr. Rodriguez is not ready for discharge. However, you are getting pressure from the Emergency Department to discharge Mr. Rodriguez, because they are backed up and desperately need the bed.

2. After your initial reaction, describe your plan of action. Identify your priority. How does your critical thinking process guide your decision?

The initial priority is to discharge Mr. Rodriguez by ensuring that he has at least the minimal information needed to administer his insulin safely. Given that extending his stay in the hospital is not an option, immediate action must be taken. The wrong decision could be harmful to Mr. Rodriguez.

You need to assess Mr. Rodriguez's comprehension about his disease process, his understanding of how to prevent complications, and his ability to self-administer his insulin. The critical thinking process not only reviews the facts of this situation but also looks at its affective and emotional side. What are some issues that may not have been considered when Mr. Rodriguez was diagnosed? What are the cultural considerations? What are the social factors that may affect how he views himself and how others in his family and social circle view him and his disease? Are there any lifestyle changes that will affect not only him but also the others in his family? The language barrier only complicates the situation. The pending discharge could result in a future readmission with complications if Mr. Rodriguez does not leave today with the proper education and understanding.

The first plan of action could be to follow the nursing process as one method of decision-making. The patient should be assessed for his current knowledge and understanding of the disease process and ways to prevent complications. Insulin administration and glucose monitoring need to be observed and assessed. Once a baseline is established, Mr. Rodriguez can be given additional information. One important point to make is that the more his family is involved; the more likely that Mr. Rodriguez will be compliant. His children, who are bilingual, can help in bridging the language gap; however, keep in mind that they are only 8 and 10 years old and should not be the primary translators.

3. Identify others who may be able to assist in your decision-making.

Many institutions have a diabetic nurse educator whose primary responsibility is the education of patients with diabetes. Your first call should be to this nurse to see if he or she can offer any assistance. There may be Spanish literature, a video in Spanish, or other materials that Mr. Rodriguez does not yet have that this nurse educator can supply. The nurse educator also may be able to come to Mr. Rodriguez and do an abbreviated teaching session. Hopefully, this scenario does not happen often, but a precedent teaching session may already in place for situations such as this.

Are there predetermined employees in the hospital who can help with the translation? Generally, these translators have to pass a test that establishes their understanding of medical terminology so that interpretation is accurate.

Finally, are there any community resources that Mr. Rodriguez can "hook" into so that he will have someone to ask questions of and someone to support him once he has been discharged? Can a visiting nurse service be contacted so that periodic visits can be made to ensure compliance and to prevent readmission because of complications? Will a community-based case manager be following Mr. Rodriguez's progress?

4. Describe some of the factors that you considered while contemplating your alternative decisions.

Two issues need to be considered almost simultaneously. First is an imminent discharge of someone who is ill-prepared to go home given the current parameters, and second is the language barrier in comprehending the teaching instructions. Alternatives are limited in this situation. Mr. Rodriguez needs to be discharged as soon as possible. At the same time, he still needs diabetic education and an assessment of his understanding and ability to self-administer medication. These two factors alone guide the quick decision-making and subsequent thought processes. Few options may be available, but where the critical thinking component comes into play is the ability to be creative while meeting the client's goals. How can you ensure that he receives diabetic teaching in a timely manner while still preparing him for discharge? How can you engage his family? Is there anyone in the community to involve, and if so, would Mr. Rodriguez accept this person? What are the cultural and social issues to consider in this case?

Case Scenario 20-2

The coronary care unit (CCU) that you manage currently has seven staff openings—more than you can ever remember—and you are unable to hire registered nurses with experience. The nurse recruiter has called you several times and asked if you would consider taking new graduates into the CCU, which until now you have always rejected, requiring at least 2 years of medical-surgical experience before transfer into the unit. Today, the Director of Critical Care calls a meeting of all the critical care managers because of the vast number of registered nurse staff openings in the division that are going unfilled. He asks all the managers to come up with a solution to the shortage of staff—and closing beds cannot be an option.

Case Considerations

1. Describe the steps the critical care managers will take in outlining their plan of action to meet the Director of Critical Care's instructions.
2. Identify the data and other information that you need to develop alternative actions.
3. Create at least five alternative actions for meeting the directive.
4. What types of tools can you use in helping the managers make the best decision? Develop one to assist the management group in weighing the different options.
5. Define several methods of group decision-making. Are all appropriate to this situation? Why, or why not? Which would you suggest be applied?
6. Describe several potential limitations in making decisions in this scenario.

Case Analysis

Staffing shortages are not new to the profession of nursing; in fact, they frequently are cyclical in nature, with several years of oversupply and several years of shortage. Among nursing management, an unwritten "rule" often exists that a nurse cannot even be considered for a staff position in a critical care area without at least 1 year of experience in a medical-surgical unit. However, with the current shortage in registered nurses and, more specifically, a more severe shortage in the nursing specialties (e.g., critical care), management is forced to consider different alternatives to safely staff the units.

■ KEY POINTS

1. When making decisions, numerous viewpoints need to be considered to arrive at the most logical alternative solutions.

2. Several instruments can assist the decision-making process by highlighting different concerns. These instruments include the decision-making grid, the PERT model, the decision tree, and the Gantt chart.
3. Group decision-making can be effective in making those decisions that affect many people. Other techniques, however, such as consensus building, encourage everyone to participate in the process.
4. When involved with a group in the decision-making process, be aware of groupthink, which occurs when members are not allowed to express their individual opinions.

Case Scenario 20-3

Examine a recent group activity in which you participated that was a challenge; this activity can be a school project or an activity that occurred with an outside interest group. The only requirements for this exercise is the situation called for a group rather than an individual decision and more than two people were in the group.

Case Considerations

1. What was the ultimate goal of the group activity? What was the final decision?
2. Why did the decision-making process require a group rather than an individual decision? What are the pros and cons to a group decision-making process?
3. How effective was the group in arriving at a decision? Identify some of the barriers to effective decision-making in a group setting.
4. Were any particular techniques used in the group decision-making process?
5. Describe any groupthink activity, and discuss how it could have been avoided.
6. Explain everyone's role in the group decision-making process.

Case Analysis

Many decisions cannot be made by an individual and require the input and assistance of others. Working effectively with groups can often become a challenge for all the members, not just for the leader of the group.

■ *KEY POINTS*

1. When making decisions, it is important to gather as many facts and data as possible so that you can make an informed decision.
2. To make a decision, do not try to collect all the information yourself. Instead, delegate this task, and have others write down what they find. The first set of data to be collected may not always yield the right information.
3. All the assembled information is reviewed. There may be information that supports one decision as well as information that supports a contrary decision. Data should be reviewed in its entirety to decrease bias and groupthink.
4. There are always pros and cons to every decision. Look at them thoughtfully before a final decision is made, and keep in mind the ramifications of the decision.
5. Sometimes, maintaining the status quo is comfortable—but it may not be the best decision to make in the end.

References

Cawthorpe, D., & Harris, D. (1999). Nominal group technique: Assessing staff concerns. *Journal of Nursing Administration, 29* (7), 11, 18, 37, 42.

Finkler, S. A., & Kovner, C. T. (2000). *Financial management for nurse managers and nurse executives* (2nd ed.). Philadelphia: W. B. Saunders.

Pesut, D. J., & Herman, J. (1999). *Clinical reasoning: The art and science of critical and creative thinking.* Clifton Park, NY: Delmar Learning.

Suggested Readings

Bass, B. (1980). *Bass and Stodgill's handbook of leadership.* New York: Free Press.

Bennis, W., & Nannus, B. (1985). *Leaders: The strategies for taking charge.* New York: Harper & Row.

Boney, J., & Baker, J. D. (1997). Strategies for teaching clinical decision-making. *Nurse Educator, 17* (1), 16–21.

Daft., R. L., & Marcic, D. (2001). *Understanding management* (3rd ed.). Philadelphia: Harcourt College.

Duschscher, J. (1999). Catching the wave: Understanding the concept of critical thinking. *Journal of Advanced Nursing, 29* (3), 577–583.

Gokerbach, V. (1995). Better decision-making: A practical model for nurse managers. *Nursing Economic$, 13* (4), 197–202.

Hammond, J. S., Keeney, R. L., & Raiffa, H. (1998). The hidden traps in decision-making. *Harvard Business Review, 76* (5), 47–58.

Jones, R. A., & Beck, S. E. (1996). *Decision-making in nursing*. Clifton Park, NY: Delmar Learning.

Kennison, M., & Bruce, J. (1997). Critical thinking: Digging deeper for creative solutions. *Nursing, 27* (9), 52–54.

Marquis, B. L., & Huston, C. J. (1998). *Management decision-making for nurses* (3rd ed.). Philadelphia: J. B. Lippincott.

Rowland, H. S., & Rowland, B. L. (1997). *Nursing administration handbook* (4th ed.). Gaithersburg, MD: Aspen Publishers.

Simms, L. M., Price, S. A., & Ervin, N. E. (2000). *Professional practice of nursing administration* (3rd ed.). Clifton Park, NY: Delmar Learning.

Vroom, V. H., & Yetton, P. W. (1973). *Leadership and decision-making*. Pittsburgh, PA: University of Pittsburgh Press.

Wolper, L. (1999). *Health care administration planning, implementing and managing organized delivery systems* (3rd ed.). Gaithersburg, MD: Aspen Publishers.

UNIT

VI

Other Professional Considerations

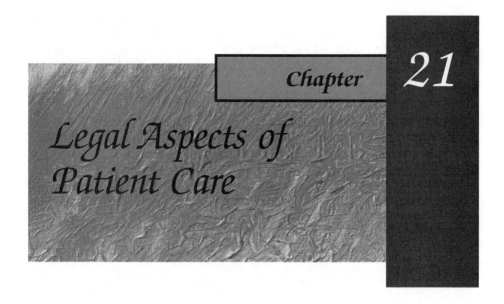

Chapter 21

Legal Aspects of Patient Care

Essential Legal Concepts of Nursing

The purpose of any law is to protect a designated population. Because of certain laws and legislation, the scope of acceptable nursing practice is defined and maintained, and safe patient care is upheld. There are two primary sources of law in the United States: public, which consists of constitutional, criminal, and administrative law; and civil, which consists mostly of contract and tort law. The practice of nursing predominately falls into the category of civil tort law, which contains the issues of negligence, malpractice, and assault and battery.

Public Law

- Public law comprises those laws that are maintained by the government to protect its citizens.
- Constitutional law encompasses the rights that someone has as an American citizen.
- Criminal law safeguards those who have been harmed. Criminal law affects nursing practice in the area of an institution performing

background criminal checks on their employees, laws that protect
the vulnerable from harm, and laws that require strict accounting of
regulated drugs.

Administrative Law

- Administrative law, like public law, protects the rights of citizens.
  Administrative law sometimes goes beyond the protections found
  in state and federal constitutions. Examples of federal agencies that
  protect the health care interest of patients and providers alike
  include the Equal Employment Opportunity Commission, the
  Occupational Safety and Health Administration, and the National
  Labor Relations Board.

Civil Law

- Civil law is the area in which nurses are more likely to be involved.
- Tort law includes actions that are both intentional and unintentional. Malpractice is often the failure of a professional to act in a
  reasonable and prudent manner. Negligence is the omission to act
  in the way that someone else in a similar situation would act.
- To prove negligence or malpractice, four generally accepted parameters must be met by the plaintiff: (1) a duty or obligation to practice
  must be established, (2) a breach of duty must be found, (3) harm
  must have occurred, and (4) harm must have occurred because of
  the omission in the duty to act.
- The most common areas in which nursing practice is involved
  include failure to monitor, assess, or communicate patient findings
  and failure to follow the standards of nursing practice. To minimize
  risk from these actions, the prudent nurse should adhere to the
  standard of accepted nursing practice for the state in which he or
  she is licensed but also be cognizant of the institution's standards of
  practice and the care in the community.
- Assault and battery occurs when a person is either threatened or
  actually touched against their will.

Advance Directives

- The living will is an instrument that delineates the specific care that
  a person desires if he or she should become unable to communicate
  while terminally ill. Federal law requires that institutions ask all
  patients if they have a living will upon admission to the hospital.

Table 21-1 Actions to Decrease the Risk of Liability

- Communicate with your clients by keeping them informed and listening to what they say.
- Acknowledge unfortunate incidents, and express concern about these events without either taking the blame, blaming others, or reacting defensively.
- Chart and time your observations immediately, while facts are still fresh in your mind.
- Take appropriate actions to meet the client's nursing needs.
- Follow the facility's policies and procedures for administering care and reporting incidents.
- Acknowledge and document the reason for any omission or deviation from agency policy, procedure, or standard.
- Maintain clinical competency, and acknowledge your limitations. If you do not know how to do something, ask for help.
- Promptly report any concern regarding the quality of care, including the lack of resources with which to provide care, to a nursing administration representative.
- Use appropriate standards of care.
- Document the time of changes in conditions requiring notification of the physician, and include the response of the physician.
- Delegate client care based on the documented skills of licensed and unlicensed personnel.
- Treat all clients and their families with kindness and respect.

- The medical power of attorney gives a designated person the right to make medical decisions on behalf of someone who is found to be incompetent.
- Do-not-resuscitate orders are written by a physician to direct the staff not to initiate cardiopulmonary resuscitation in the event of a sudden cardiopulmonary arrest.

The Role of Risk Management

- To protect the interest of the patient, the health care provided, and the institution, risk management programs are designed to quickly recognize and rectify potential problem situations.
- Risk management uses the techniques of quality improvement to protect the institution from financial liability.
- The Risk Management Department generally maintains the responsibility of tracking incident reports that are filed in the institution.
- Actions to decrease the risk of liability are outlined in Table 21-1.

CASE SCENARIOS

Guided Case Scenario 21-1

One morning, you are making rounds on your presurgical patients when you stop in to see Mrs. Guo, who you have listed as undergoing a bilateral salpingo-oophorectomy and hysterectomy later in the day. Her new husband of 3 months has stopped in to see her before he goes to work and is planning to come back to the hospital after her surgery. English is not their primary language, and both struggle to communicate with you.

They both appear to be anxious, but they obviously are very much in love. When you comment on this, they both say that they waited a long time to get married because of Mrs. Guo's illness but that once this surgery is over, they can move on to begin a family.

Case Considerations

1. Identify your first thoughts and response.
2. What is the primary issue here?
3. Describe the course of action that should be taken at this point, and provide your rationale.
4. Discuss the legal ramifications of several possible decisions, including doing nothing.

Case Analysis

1. Identify your first thoughts and response.

   The first thought would be to question the patient's understanding of her pending surgery. Obviously, there is a disconnect between the surgery that she is assuming she will have and what the surgeon intends to do. This disconnect can be caused by several factors. Is there a language barrier between the physician and the patient? Did the physician clearly explain the surgery and the outcomes of the surgery? Did the physician even attempt to explain the surgery and the outcomes to the patient? Does the patient understand the surgery and the outcomes?

2. What is the primary issue here?

   There appears to be an issue with informed consent. Generally, informed consent requires that two primary criteria are satisfied. The first criterion is that the person giving consent must fully comprehend the procedure; in other words, the risks of doing the procedure, the projected outcomes, the potential complications, and any alternative therapies that could be administered instead of the given procedure are explained and understood. The second criterion is that the person who gives consent has the legal authority to do so.

In this case, Mrs. Guo clearly does not understand the procedure that she is about to undergo, its risks, its projected outcomes, and its possible complications. It is the responsibility of the physician to obtain informed consent by explaining the procedure in terms that the patient can understand. The physician needs to describe the procedure, the risks, the projected outcome, and the possible alternatives to having surgery. All of this is done while assuming that the patient is competent. Only a competent adult can sign the informed consent form for procedures. Several situations may be considered if an adult is not competent to sign. A legal guardian, or one who has been appointed by the court, can sign for the patient. A parent can sign for a child. An emancipated or married minor or a minor themselves may also be able to sign, given a particular situation. In addition, an emergency situation invokes implied consent. For example, an unconscious patient who is brought into the Emergency Department by ambulance will receive care even though that patient cannot give informed consent.

3. Describe the course of action that should be taken at this point, and provide your rationale.

   At this point, the best alternative would be to call the physician immediately and detail the conversation that you just had with the Guos. Obviously, as the patient's advocate, there is a concern that Mrs. Guo does not understand the procedure and its ramifications. Before the patient is premedicated, the physician needs to ensure that he has clearly explained the procedure to Mrs. Guo—even though he may have to delay the case while waiting for an interpreter.

4. Discuss the legal ramifications of several possible decisions, including doing nothing.

   As the nurse assigned to this case, you have several alternative actions to consider. The first is to inform the physician of your findings. This alternative is the most appropriate—and the most correct—both ethically and legally. A second alternative is to attempt to clarify the information for the Guos yourself, including teaching them about the procedure, its risks, and its projected outcomes. This alternative is in opposition to their understanding of the procedure, however, and it may contradict information given by the physician, which may place you in a legal situation. The final alternative is to do nothing, letting Mrs. Guo have the surgery under false pretenses, which is ethically and morally the incorrect decision.

Case Scenario 21-2

Today has been an especially busy shift because the unit is short staffed. As the team leader for 12 pediatric patients, you have taken the responsibility for medication administration for the entire team. After giving Baby Harris his medications, you realize that instead of administering 0.025 mg IVP of Digoxin, you mistakenly administered 0.25 mg IVP.

Case Considerations

1. Describe the legal situation at hand.
2. What is the first action to take in this situation, and why?
3. Define your alternative actions, and describe the ramifications of your actions.
4. Discuss the nurse's negligence and liability in this scenario.

Case Analysis

Incorrect medication administration is one of the most common sources of liability for nurses. Administering medication has potential to be the most dangerous action that a nurse can perform, yet many times, despite the responsibility to perform the five rights of medication on each patient, patients still receive the wrong medication, the wrong dose, the wrong route, or have the medication administered regardless of known contraindications.

■ KEY POINTS

1. Nursing care standards of practice include understanding the medication that is administered, including its actions, side effects, and contraindications.
2. Nurses are expected to use their judgment with medication orders and administration. Questioning an order that is written

poorly, that has the wrong dosage, or that is contraindicated is always appropriate as a nursing action.
3. The nurse needs to be familiar with the institution's policies and procedures for medication administration.
4. Once a medication is administered, the nurse needs to document this accurately and in a timely manner. Any side effects of the medication also need to be documented.
5. Often, medication errors are made because of haste in administration. Taking the time to read the labels of the medications and checking against the medication administration record and the order sets usually decrease the rate of errors.
6. Always assess the patient for known effects of the medication, and know when to notify the physician if side effects occur.
7. Do not administer a medication at a dosage that you feel may be incorrect. Always validate a questionable dosage with the person who wrote the order. A pharmacist may also be able to assist you with correct dosages.
8. Once a medication is given incorrectly, understand your legal responsibilities to the patient and what actions need to be taken.

Case Scenario 21-3

As a nursing student, you are required to carry malpractice insurance. When you graduate and go into practice as a registered nurse, the decision to carry malpractice insurance is no longer a requirement, unless you are acting in a specialized role, such as a nurse anesthetist, nurse practitioner, or nurse midwife.

Case Considerations

1. What is the purpose of carrying malpractice insurance for registered nurses?
2. Does the employing agency always carry malpractice insurance for its professional employees?
3. Identify the pros for carrying personal malpractice insurance for registered nurses.
4. Identify the cons for carrying personal malpractice insurance for registered nurses.
5. Discuss the items you should look for in a personal malpractice policy for registered nurses.
6. Describe the amounts most commonly covered under a personal malpractice policy for registered nurses.

7. Where would you purchase personal malpractice insurance for registered nurses?

Case Analysis

Purchasing malpractice insurance is a personal decision, with many people having differing opinions. It is much more common for physicians to carry malpractice insurance—it is actually a requirement—than it is for nurses. Part of the reason why not all registered nurses carry malpractice insurance is history: Nurses have not, historically, been charged in as many lawsuits as physicians, and fewer companies insure nurses. Whatever the case, nurses often waver between carrying their own policies or counting on their employer's policy to cover them if they ever are called to court.

■ KEY POINTS

1. For the coverage obtained, malpractice insurance for nonspecialty registered nurses is relatively inexpensive.
2. In the litigious atmosphere of today's society, it is prudent for the professional nurse to understand fully the ramifications of declining to carry personal malpractice insurance.
3. Some malpractice policies can be tailored to meet an individual nurse's needs.
4. Issues must be clearly defined when considering whether to carry individual malpractice insurance or employer-sponsored coverage.

Suggested Readings

Aiken, T. D. (1994). *Legal, ethical, and political issues in nursing.* Philadelphia: F. A. Davis.

Fiesta, J. (1999). Do no harm: When caregivers violate our golden rule, part 1. *Nursing Management, 30* (8), 10–11.

Fiesta, J. (1999). Informed consent: What health care professionals need to know, part 1. *Nursing Management, 30* (6), 8–9.

Fiesta, J. (1999). Informed consent: What health care professionals need to know, part 2. *Nursing Management, 30* (7), 6–7.

Guido, G. (1988). *Legal issues in nursing: A sourcebook for practice.* Norwalk, CT: Appleton & Lange.

Laben, J. K., & Rudolph, E. G. (1997). Nursing case law update: ERISA and state statutes relating to professional liability: A complex maze. *Journal of Nursing Law, 4* (2), 59–63.

LaDuke, S. (2000). What should you expect from your attorney? *Nursing Management, 31* (1), 10.

Marquis, B. L., & Huston, C. J. (2000). *Leadership roles and management functions* (3rd ed.). Philadelphia: J. B. Lippincott.

Olsen-Chavarriaga, D. (2000). Informed consent: Do you know your role? *Nursing 2000, 30* (5), 60–61.

Rowland, H. S., & Rowland, B. L. (1997). *Nursing administration handbook* (4th ed.). Gaithersburg, MD: Aspen Publishers.

Simms, L. M., Price, S. A., & Ervin, N. E. (2000). *Professional practice of nursing administration* (3rd ed.). Clifton Park, NY: Delmar Learning.

Smith-Pittman, M. H. (1997). Nursing and the corporate negligence doctrine. *Journal of Nursing Law, 4* (2), 41–50.

Chapter 22

Ethical Dimensions of Patient Care

Essential Concepts of Ethical Nursing Care

Nursing is perhaps one of the most intimate of all professions and therefore calls for ethical consideration of the people under our care. On a daily basis, nurses in all types of settings are confronted with ethical dilemmas, and it is imperative that they be aware of the many ethical principles that can guide decision-making. Ethical dilemmas occur when there are two or more options for an outcome—but all the choices are undesirable. An ethical decision calls for weighing the circumstances compared to the potential outcomes.

Numerous issues come into play when attempting to make an ethical decision, including personal values and morals, beliefs and philosophies, and even institutional guidelines. Ethical principles include those of beneficence, nonmaleficence, justice, autonomy, fidelity, respect for others, veracity, and many more. Often, when an institution has to make a difficult ethical decision, it will call a meeting of the ethics committee, which is comprised of a variety of individuals. Through these individual belief sets, many aspects of the patient's circumstance are considered. Regardless of the outcome, all ethical dilemmas require critical thinking and the ability to evaluate right from wrong decisions.

Ethics

- Ethics are statements of what is right or wrong, or what should be, in concert with one's morals, values, and beliefs.

Ethical Principles and Theories as the Basis for Nursing Practice

- Teleology, which is also called Utilitarianism, states that an individual situation determines whether an outcome is determined to be morally right or wrong. The effects of alternative actions are weighted in making decisions (Aiken, 1994).
- Deontology is focused on the moral rules that govern a society and the principles that assist in decision-making. The outcomes of the act are not as crucial as the motives of the person (Aiken, 1994).
- Clinical practice in nursing is based on numerous ethical principles, including beneficence, nonmaleficence, justice, autonomy, fidelity, respect, and veracity.

Participation on the Ethics Committee

- With the ethical dilemmas facing patients and health care providers alike, the hospital ethics committee offers nurses, physicians, administrators, and patients decision-making assistance. Ethics committees are interdisciplinary in nature. They include representatives from clinical services, clergy, legal and risk management services, and the community.

Burkhardt and Nathaniel's Guide for Decision-Making

- Situations often present themselves as ethical dilemmas, and it is helpful to have a guide to follow when making decisions.
- The key points to Burkhardt and Nathaniel's Guide for Decision-Making (Burkhardt & Nathaniel, 2002) include obtaining all the data that identify the moral conflict, those that are creating the conflict, the moral perspectives, the options, and the desired outcomes. Once a decision to act is made, then the actual outcome is evaluated.

Ethical Issues Surrounding Nursing Practice

- Providing nursing care is sometimes made more complex when various issues come into consideration that can cause moral distress. Issues such as cost-containment initiatives, the application and continuation of technology, and the application of the American Hospital Association's Patient's Bill of Rights (1992) can all lead to the nurse being faced with difficult decisions. Nurses are held accountable for upholding the Patient's Bill of Rights (Table 22-1).

- Sometimes, a nurse may struggle with decisions that are made and with orders that are given by a physician. Institutional policies can often assist the nurse with his or her decision strategy. Resources may include the ethics committee, an ethics team, and perhaps, even assistance from the clergy working with the patient.

Table 22-1 A Patient's Bill of Rights

Introduction

Effective health care requires collaboration between patients and physicians and other health care professionals. Open and honest communication, respect for personal and professional values, and sensitivity to differences are integral to optimal patient care. As the setting for the provision of health services, hospitals must provide a foundation for understanding and respecting the rights and responsibilities of patients, their families, physicians, and other caregivers. Hospitals must ensure a health care ethic that respects the role of patients in decision making about treatment choices and other aspects of their care. Hospitals must be sensitive to cultural, racial, linguistic, religious, age, gender, and other differences as well as the needs of persons with disabilities.

The American Hospital Association presents *A Patient's Bill of Rights* with the expectation that it will contribute to more effective patient care and be supported by the hospital on behalf of the institution, its medical staff, employees, and patients. The American Hospital Association encourages health care institutions to tailor this bill of rights to their patient community by translating and/or simplifying the language of this bill as may be necessary to ensure that patients and their families understand their rights and responsibilities.

Bill of Rights*

1. The patient has the right to considerate and respectful care.
2. The patient has the right to and is encouraged to obtain from physicians and other direct caregivers relevant, current, and understandable information concerning diagnosis, treatment, and prognosis. Except in emergencies when the patient lacks decision-making capacity and the need for treatment is urgent, the patient is entitled to the opportunity to discuss and request information related to the specific procedures and/or treatments, the risks involved, the possible length of recuperation, and the medically reasonable alternatives and their accompanying risks and benefits. Patients have the right to know the identity of physicians, nurses, and others involved in their care, as well as when those involved are students, residents, or other trainees. The patient also has the right to know the immediate and long-term financial implications of treatment choices, insofar as they are known.

(Table continues on following page.)

3. The patient has the right to make decisions about the plan of care prior to and during the course of treatment and to refuse a recommended treatment or plan of care to the extent permitted by law and hospital policy and to be informed of the medical consequences of this action. In case of such refusal, the patient is entitled to other appropriate care and services that the hospital provides or transfer to another hospital. The hospital should notify patients of any policy that might affect patient choice within the institution.

4. The patient has the right to have an advance directive (such as a living will, health care proxy, or durable power of attorney for health care) concerning treatment or designating a surrogate decision maker with the expectation that the hospital will honor the intent of that directive to the extent permitted by law and hospital policy. Health care institutions must advise patients of their rights under state law and hospital policy to make informed medical choices, ask if the patient has an advance directive, and include that information in patient records. The patient has the right to timely information about hospital policy that may limit its ability to implement fully a legally valid advance directive.

5. The patient has the right to every consideration of privacy. Case discussion, consultation, examination, and treatment should be conducted so as to protect each patient's privacy.

6. The patient has the right to expect that all communications and records pertaining to his/her care will be treated as confidential by the hospital, except in cases such as suspected abuse and public health hazards when reporting is permitted or required by law. The patient has the right to expect that the hospital will emphasize the confidentiality of this information when it releases it to any other parties entitled to review information in these records.

7. The patient has the right to review the records pertaining to his/her medical care and to have the information explained or interpreted as necessary, except when restricted by law.

8. The patient has the right to expect that, within its capacity and policies, a hospital will make reasonable response to the request of a patient for appropriate and medically indicated care and services. The hospital must provide evaluation, service, and/or referral as indicated by the urgency of the case. When medically appropriate and legally permissible, or when a patient has so requested, a patient may be transferred to another facility. The institution to which the patient is to be transferred must first have accepted the patient for transfer. The patient must also have the benefit of complete information and explanation concerning the need for, risks, benefits, and alternatives to such a transfer.

9. The patient has the right to ask and be informed of the existence of business relationships among the hospital, educational institutions, other health care providers, or payers that may influence the patient's treatment and care.

10. The patient has the right to consent to or decline to participate in proposed research studies or human experimentation affecting care and treatment or requiring direct patient involvement, and to have those studies fully explained prior to consent. A patient who declines to participate in research

or experimentation is entitled to the most effective care that the hospital can otherwise provide.

11. The patient has the right to expect reasonable continuity of care when appropriate and to be informed by physicians and other caregivers of available and realistic patient care options when hosptial care is no longer appropriate.

12. The patient has the right to be informed of hospital policies and practices that relate to patient care, treatment, and responsibilities. The patient has the right to be informed of available resources for resolving disputes, grievances, and conflicts, such as ethics committees, patient representatives, or other mechanisms available in the institution. The patient has the right to be informed of the hospital's charges for services and available payment methods.

The collaborative nature of health care requires that patients, or their families/ surrogates, participate in their care. The effectiveness of care and patient satisfaction with the course of treatment depend, in part, on the patient fulfilling certain responsibilities. Patients are responsible for providing information about past illnesses, hospitalizations, medications, and other matters related to health status. To participate effectively in decision making, patients must be encouraged to take responsibility for requesting additional information or clarification about their health status or treatment when they do not fully understand information and instructions. Patients are also responsible for ensuring that the health care institution has a copy of their written advance directive if they have one. Patients are responsible for informing their physicians and other caregivers if they anticipate problems in following prescribed treatment.

Patients should also be aware of the hospital's obligation to be reasonably efficient and equitable in providing care to other patients and the community. The hospital's rules and regulations are designed to help the hospital meet this obligation. Patients and their families are responsible for making reasonable accommodations to the needs of the hospital, other patients, medical staff, and hospital employees. Patients are responsible for providing necessary information for insurance claims and for working with the hospital to make payment arrangements, when necessary.

A person's health depends on much more than health care services. Patients are responsible for recognizing the impact of their life-style on their personal health.

Conclusion

Hospitals have many functions to perform, including the enhancement of health status, health promotion, and the prevention and treatment of injury and disease; the immediate and ongoing care and rehabilitation of patients; the education of health professionals, patients, and the community; and research. All these activities must be conducted with an overriding concern for the values and dignity of patients.

*These rights can be exercised on the patient's behalf by a designated surrogate or proxy decision maker if the patient lacks decision-making capacity, is legally incompetent, or is a minor.

A Patient's Bill of Rights was first adopted by the American Hospital Association in 1973. This revision was approved by the AHA Board of Trustees on October 21, 1992. Copyright 1992 by the American Hospital Association, 840 North Lake Short Drive, Chicago, IL 60611. Printed in the U.S.A. All rights reserved. Reprinted with permission of the American Hospital Association.

CASE SCENARIOS

Guided Case Scenario 22-1

For the last few days, you have been taking care of Mr. Cole, a 28-year-old patient with end-stage cystic fibrosis. You have developed a caring relationship with Mr. Cole and his wife. They are both aware of the prognosis of his disease, and they realize that he only has a short time to live.

When Dr. Xui made rounds with you this morning, she told the Coles that Mr. Cole could be discharged today if his condition remains stable. Mr. and Mrs. Cole were both excited about the news, because they have been urging the doctor to let him go home to enjoy his remaining time surrounded by the things and the people he loves.

When you bring Mr. Cole's discharge orders to his room to review his medications and other treatments, you find Mrs. Cole assisting Mr. Cole as he coughs up bright-red blood. When you come to them, they both beg you not to tell the doctor or chart the incident. They believe it is their right to go home and let Mr. Cole die surrounded by his family. They said they know they can leave AMA (against medical advice), but if they do, their insurance will not pay for home care.

Case Considerations

1. Describe the duty of the professional nurse in this case with Mr. Cole.
2. Discuss Mr. Cole's rights as a patient. Should they figure into your decision?
3. Is it ever justified to knowingly withhold patient information from a physician? Why, or why not?
4. Identify and discuss several ethical principles and guidelines that will assist and justify your decision.
5. Will you chart the incident, and will you report it to anyone?

Case Analysis

1. Describe the duty of the professional nurse in this case with Mr. Cole.

   Duty is described as the responsibility to the patient under the care of a professional. Once a relationship has been initiated, the professional has a duty to continue the relationship until it is completed or another professional can be substituted. In this scenario, the registered nurse has a duty to provide nursing care for Mr. Cole using appropriate standards of practice. Duty-based reasoning is an ethical framework that can be applied in this case. In duty-based reasoning, a decision can be made because of the relationship between the person with the duty to act (e.g., the professional nurse in this case) and the receiving person.

2. Discuss Mr. Cole's rights as a patient. Should they figure into your decision?

    The American Hospital Association (1992) has a formal Patient's Bill of Rights to which all hospitals subscribe, many of them with formal policies in place for the protection of the patient. Clearly, Mr. Cole has several rights, including the right to "considerate and respectful care"; the right to "relevant, current and understandable information concerning diagnosis, treatment and prognosis"; the right to "make decisions about the plan of care prior and during the course of treatment and to refuse a recommended treatment"; the right to have an advance directive; the right to privacy and confidentiality; the right to review relevant hospital records; and others (Kelly-Heidenthal, in Little, 2003, pp. 473–474).

    Knowing that Mr. Cole has these rights, the nurse is presented with an ethical dilemma: whether to inform Mr. Cole's physician, against his wishes, that he is having symptoms that may cause him to extend his stay in the hospital. How do Mr. Cole's rights factor into what would be best practice, both in medical and in nursing care? Remember, an ethical dilemma is one in which all the outcomes are undesirable, forcing one to chose between them.

3. Is it ever justified to knowingly withhold patient information from a physician? Why, or why not?

    It is never justifiable to withhold information from the physician. Accurate communication of patient care information, whether written or verbally, to members of the health care team is imperative. By withholding information from a physician, especially information as critical as Mr. Cole's bleeding, the nurse may be held personally liable for negligence or malpractice.

4. Identify and discuss several ethical principles and guidelines that will assist and justify your decision.

Several ethical principles and guidelines can assist the nurse with decision-making in this scenario. Beneficence is a principle that applies here, in that the nurse has a duty to provide the best care to the patient. Nonmaleficence, or the principle of doing no harm, also applies, because the patient could potentially be harmed if the nurse does not make the physician aware of Mr. Cole's bleeding.

Two other ethical principles that would be appropriate to apply to the decision-making process would be those of autonomy and advocacy. Respecting a patient's decision to self-determination is legally established by the court systems in a variety of venues, most frequently with right-to-die legislation. Autonomy involves more than self-determination, however, because it also includes respecting the patient's privacy, not discussing their information with others who are not professionally involved with them, and ensuring that consent is obtained for all tests and procedures. The last ethical principle to consider when deciding whether to inform the physician of Mr. Cole's bleeding is that of respect for others—or the right of people to make their own decision. In this particular case, Mr. Cole has the right to go home, but he needs to have all the information about the possible side effects of his bleeding, what ramifications his actions will have on his quality of life, and the ability of the physician and other health care team members to provide for him the best possible care.

5. Will you chart the incident, and will you report it to anyone?

This is a highly personal decision and is fraught with potential dangers if the correct choice—let alone the most ethical decision—is not made. If the nurse does not inform the physician and discharges Mr. Cole, then how can a discharge summary be written truthfully? What if Mr. Cole begins severely bleeding once he is home, requiring an emergency admittance to the hospital, and he states that he actually began bleeding in the hospital before he was discharged? What would the nurse's liability (as well as the physician's) be at that point? Many nurses treat their patients empathetically, but it is necessary to remember that the primary responsibility of nurses is ensuring that a patient is cared for to the best of their abilities.

Case Scenario 22-2

A licensed practical nurse (LPN) comes to you, her team leader, and says that she came across a disturbing situation in

Mr. Thompson's room while doing rounds. As you review the Kardex on Mr. Thompson, you read that he was admitted 3 days ago for dehydration and severe weight loss during the last few months. He also has prostate cancer, for which he was unsuccessfully treated.

Mr. Thompson was seen throwing his food into the garbage can without eating anything from his tray. When the LPN went into the top drawer of his bedside table to retrieve his glasses, which he could not find, she also found numerous pills that he supposedly had taken during the last few days. When she asked why the pills were in the drawer, he said that he did not want to take them, because they "won't help anymore."

Case Considerations

1. Define the ethical dilemma in this scenario. Why is it an ethical dilemma? What is the underlying issue, and why has it become an issue?
2. Identify at least three ethical principles that could possibly assist you and the LPN in solving their ethical dilemma with Mr. Thompson. What in particular could potentially guide your decision?
3. Name several morals, belief sets, or values that appear to be in conflict with the nursing staff that led to the dilemma.
4. Are there any legal issues to be concerned with in Mr. Thompson's case? How do the legal ramifications affect the ethical issues in this scenario?
5. Is Mr. Thompson competent? How would someone assess his status? Why does competency have any bearing on the dilemma's outcome? Can a competent person refuse to eat? Refuse medications? Refuse treatments?
6. Discuss several options that may be possibilities in this case. Which would be the best outcome, and why?

Case Analysis

When a patient refuses to eat or take his or her medications, regardless of age, it is always a distressing situation for the professional caregiver, who wants to assist the patient in the best way possible. Many cultures equate living with food and hydration, so it is particularly hard to see someone refuse nutrition.

■ KEY POINTS

1. The first step when confronted with an ethical dilemma is to identify the issue clearly.

2. After clearly identifying the issue or problem, distinguish the morals, values, and beliefs sets. Which of them are in conflict?
3. Next, review as much information about the particular situation as possible, because surrounding circumstances often contribute to the dilemma itself and therefore must be considered as well.
4. Others who may be involved on the case are then sought for their insight and possible solutions. Do they all see the dilemma in the same light, or do their opinions differ?
5. Once all the data are in and have been discussed, a choice or decision needs to be reached. Again, with an ethical dilemma, all the options may be unfavorable; however, a choice does need to be made about the outcome.

Case Scenario 22-3

Mrs. Ling has been a patient in the neurosciences intensive care unit for more than a week after suffering a severe stroke at home that has left her comatose and unable to communicate. She is ventilator dependent and on numerous medications just to maintain her blood pressure. Today, she experienced a long run of ventricular tachycardia, and she no longer responds to stimulation. The primary physician on her case deems her progress as dim and her quality of life as poor at best.

Mrs. Ling immigrated to the United States 20 years ago; however, her English has remained quite limited. She did agree at her last doctor's visit to sign a set of advance directives, not wanting to be a burden on her growing family, and even signed that she did not want to be maintained on life support if she should have no hope for a quality life.

Her two sons and one daughter come into the room after their mother's last setback and talk with the physician, who explains the grim prognosis. The physician recommendation is to consider placing a do-not-resuscitate (DNR) status on Mrs. Ling. The children refuse to carry out Mrs. Ling's wishes; they refuse the DNR order. The children are her closest living relatives.

Case Considerations

1. How are DNR orders obtained? Who has the power to suggest them? Who can write them? Can they be overturned, and if so, how?

2. Discuss the ramifications of DNR orders? What are the parameters of care when a patient has such an order on his or her chart? Are there varying degrees of DNR orders?
3. Define the ethical dilemma in this case. What is the underlying issue, and why has it become an issue?
4. Identify several ethical principles that surround DNR orders. Which can assist the nurse and other health care team members in arriving at the best solution for Mrs. Ling?
5. Name several morals, belief sets, or values that appear to be in conflict with those involved with Mrs. Ling's care.
6. Are there any legal issues to be concerned with in Mrs. Ling's situation? How do the legal ramifications affect the ethical issues in this scenario?
7. Would the Ethics Committee be helpful in this situation? Discuss the purpose of the Ethics Committee. What steps would the committee take if it reviewed this case? Identify the type of guidance the committee could offer to the staff, the physician, and to the family.

Case Analysis

One of the most difficult situations a nurse may face is when a patient's prognosis is so grim that a DNR order is suggested to the family and the patient. By Mrs. Ling's signing of her advance directive, she has indicated her desire not to be maintained on life support mechanisms, such as ventilator support, medication support, and possibly, even food and hydration. This case becomes more complex because of the personal desires of her two children, who are at odds with their mother's wishes and, unfortunately for her, have the need to keep her on life support, regardless of her prognosis and quality of life.

■ KEY POINTS

1. Ideally, advance directives are first discussed in the physician's office before a patient is admitted to the hospital. It is much easier to make these serious decisions about care if the added pressures of hospitalization are not imminent.
2. Advance directives contain many pieces of information not only for the physician and other health team members but also for a patient's family. Advance directives are the patient's right to practice self-determination. Specifically, an advance directive specifies the type and intensity of care that a patient desires

should he or she become incompetent and unable sign an informed consent. Many people state their desires not to be maintained on life support should they become terminally ill, and they may even specify detailed situations and treatments.

3. When signing an advance directive, it is critically important that what is contained in the document be shared with family and others who may be acting on behalf of the patient so that everyone knows what the patient's wishes are before an unfortunate circumstance. Letting everyone know what your wishes are does not guarantee compliance if the situation arises, but at least there is be an opportunity to discuss the contents before the situation.

4. It is important to understand competency when reviewing a patient's advance directive status, ensuring that they were written during a period of lucidity and awareness.

5. If there are conflicts with the DNR order, an Ethics Committee may be helpful in offering guidance. Anyone can contact an Ethics Committee, including nurses, physicians, and family members, when a disagreement arises over the treatment plans or when members of the health care team and family cannot reach a difficult decision.

References

Aiken, T. D. (1994). *Legal, ethical and political issues in nursing.* Philadelphia: F. A. Davis.

American Hospital Association. (1992). *A patient's bill of rights.* Chicago: Author.

Burkhardt, M. A., & Nathaniel, A. K. (2002). *Ethics and issues in contemporary nursing* (2nd ed.). Clifton Park, NY: Delmar Learning.

Little, C. B. (2003). *Ethical dimensions of patient care.* In P. Kelly-Heidenthal (Ed.), Nursing leadership and management. Clifton Park, NY: Delmar Learning.

Suggested Readings

Aiken, T. D. (2002). *Legal, ethical and political issues in health occupations.* Philadelphia: F. A. Davis.

American Nurses Association. (1995). *Code for nurses with interpretative statements.* Washington, D.C.: American Nurses Publishing.

American Nurses Association. (1995). *Standards of clinical nursing practice.* Washington, D.C.: American Nurses Publishing.

Bosek, M. (1999). Bioethics in practice. *JONA's Healthcare Law, Ethics and Regulation, 1* (3), 16–19.

Edge, R. S., & Groves, J. R. (1999). *Ethics of healthcare: A guide for clinical practice* (2nd ed.). Clifton Park, NY: Delmar Learning.

Hall, J. (1996). *Nursing ethics and law.* Philadelphia: J. B. Lippincott.

Lowell, J., & Massey, K. (1997). Sounds of silence. *Nursing Management, 28* (5), 40H, 40J.

Marquis, B. L., & Huston, C. J. (1998). *Management decision making for nurses* (3rd ed.). Philadelphia: Lippincott-Raven.

Marquis, B. L., & Huston, C. J. (2000). *Leadership roles and management functions* (3rd ed.). Philadelphia: Lippincott-Raven.

Raines, M. L. (2000). Ethical decision making in nurses: Relationships among moral reasoning, coping style and ethics stress. *JONA's Healthcare Law, Ethics and Regulation, 2* (1), 29–40.

Rowland, H. S., & Rowland, B. L. (1997). *Nursing administration handbook* (4th ed.). Gaithersburg, MD: Aspen Publisher.

Simms, L. M., Price, S. A., & Ervin, N. E. (2000). *Professional practice of nursing administration* (3rd ed.). Clifton Park, NY: Delmar Learning.

Veatch, R. M., & Fry, S. T. (1987). *Case studies in nursing ethics.* Philadelphia: J. B. Lippincott.

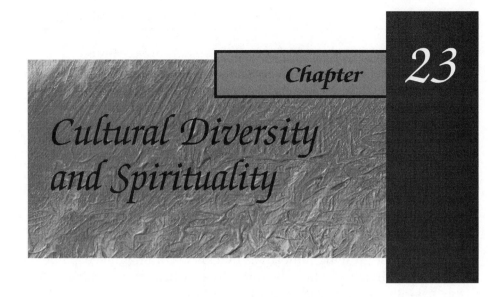

Chapter 23

Cultural Diversity and Spirituality

Essential Concepts in Cultural Diversity and Spirituality

Many places of work are becoming increasingly diverse in their composition of employees, not only in terms of gender and race but also in terms of culture and ethnicity. As a member of the health care team, the registered nurse (RN) must be able to provide culturally sensitive care to a variety of people with varying backgrounds, experiences, and expectations and to work alongside those from different backgrounds. Even those from the same cultural environment or region of the country may have different expectations based on past experiences and their personal values and belief sets.

Like culture, race, and ethnicity, religious and spiritual beliefs are interwoven into a person's personality and can affect immensely how one views health care, health care providers, and potential treatments. It is necessary that the nurse not only understand but also value those differences between patients and coworkers alike. Through appreciation of these differences, one can learn to understand the actions and behaviors of others.

Culture Defined

- Culture is based on the common beliefs, values, and behaviors of a defined community of people.
- Ethnicity evolves as people's perceptions of who they are and whom they identify with as a group change. Ethnocentrism is the belief that your culture is superior to others. Race is the grouping of a specific people based on certain biological attributes.

American Diversity

- The United States has a diverse mix of cultures, races, and ethnicities. Historically, the population has been a Caucasian majority, but the fastest-growing minority is quickly becoming the Hispanic community. In many cities, the minority cultures are becoming the majority cultures, with almost 50% of the American cultural mix in 2080 estimated to be minority ethnic groups (U.S. Bureau of the Census, 1990).
- Unfortunately, the racial and ethnic mix of health care providers does not mirror that of the population. Only approximately 10% of the nurses in the United States are from a minority background, with physicians having about the same percentage of providers who are considered to be minorities.
- The many ways in which people differ are illustrated in Figure 23-1.

Cultural Theorists

- Leininger (1997) is considered to be the founder of transcultural nursing theory. She began her studies of transcultural nursing in the 1960s, focusing on the world's different cultures and how they respond to caring behaviors, nursing care and health-illness values, and beliefs and patterns of behavior. The goal of any nurse who applies Leininger's theory is to provide culture-specific nursing care to the patient. Leininger emphasized that a practicing nurse should study each culture's lifestyle patterns, symbols, rituals, and caring behaviors.
- The Transcultural Assessment Model of Giger and Davidhizer (1999) offers the nurse a culturally sensitive tool with which to perform a patient assessment. Six concepts are described in the Transcultural Assessment Model: communication, space, social organization, time, environmental control, and biological variations.
- Campinha-Bacote (1994) identifies four elements necessary to providing culturally competent care: cultural awareness, cultural knowledge, cultural skill, and the cultural encounter.

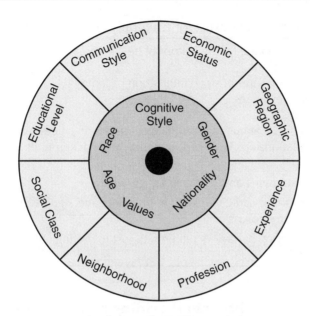

Figure 23-1   Ways in Which People Differ.

- Spector (2000) has incorporated three categories into her Cultural Heritage Model: culture, religion, and ethnicity. She also expands on some of the theoretical work by Giger and Davidhizer, incorporating space, time, communication, biological variations, social organization, and environmental control into her model to assist the nurse in performing a cultural assessment. Assessments include not only the patient but also the primary and extended family members.

Providing Culturally Competent Care

- A manager's responsibility is to ensure that patients receive the highest-quality nursing care, which includes culturally competent care.
- Understanding a patient's health beliefs provides insight regarding how he or she views health, illness, and the expectations of the health care provider.
- Applying one of the cultural assessment tools to further comprehend a patient and his or her family assists the nurse in assessing a patient's extent of family support, ability to access community resources, level of education, and level of stress as it relates to illness. These concepts lead to potentiating the optimal outcomes for the patient.
- A nursing checklist for culturally sensitive care is provided in Table 23-1.

Table 23-1   Nursing Checklist for Culturally Sensitive Care

1. Assess and incorporate family history of health care:
   - Fluency in English
   - Extent of family support or disintegration of family
   - Community resources
   - Level of education
   - Change of social status as a result of coming to this country
   - Intimate relationships with people of different backgrounds
   - Level of stress
2. Affirm client strengths and potential for growth.
3. Recognize informal caregivers (family members and significant others) as an integral part of treatment.
4. Demonstrate caring behaviors rather than just tolerating cultural variations in client's behavior.

Integrating Spirituality into Providing Nursing Care

- A critical factor to consider when providing holistic care is to incorporate a patient's spiritual or religious beliefs into the plan of care.
- Spiritual distress is a nursing diagnosis that includes a person questioning the purpose and meaning of life. Spiritual distress often occurs during a conflict between a person's religious beliefs and a particular situation or the person's desires.
- If a nurse does not feel comfortable in addressing a patient's religious viewpoints, other personnel within the health care system, such as the hospital chaplain, can be called. Nurses should not assume that because someone professes to be a member of a certain religious group that he or she personally holds all the same belief sets and values. Like the cultural assessment, a spiritual assessment should be individualized, with questions being asked rather than answers being assumed.

CASE SCENARIOS

Guided Case Scenario 23-1

After recently relocating to Miami, Florida, from Tennessee, you have taken a job as the manager of a 42-bed medical-surgical unit in a large medical center downtown. You have been an RN for more than 20 years, and you have more than 15 years of management experience. This is the first time, however, that you have worked in a large medical center with so many employees who do not have English as their first language; in fact, for many, it seems that Spanish is their first language. As a Caucasian, you feel like you are in the minority. Communication with your staff has become a barrier to effective care expectations.

Of the issues that you encounter, communication and personal values appear to be those areas giving you the most difficulty. As you begin to evaluate patient care delivery, you realize that not everyone has the same work expectations that you do, nor do they work in the same way or have the same priorities as your previous staffs. Although the staff appears pleased to have you as their manager, you are still viewed as an outsider and therefore are not included in many discussions and decisions in which you would like to partake.

Case Considerations

1. Discuss some of the cultural misperceptions that may occur because of differing styles of communication.
2. Discuss some of the steps that you, as the manager, need to take to better understand your employees.
3. What can you do to help your employees understand your cultural background and communication style?

Case Analysis

1. Discuss some of the cultural misperceptions that may occur because of differing styles of communication.

   In many areas of the country, minority populations are quickly becoming the majority population, and the workforce in health care institutions reflects these changes. Issues of communication, expectations, and values can result in conflict when a staff is multicultural and understanding of each other's culture is minimal. Those who live and work in America's larger cities often experience this increasing diversity long before those in smaller communities. As the United States continues to attract immigrants from all over the world, however, even the smallest cities are changing.

   One of the biggest issues in differing language and communication styles is that of misperception and misunderstanding. Being different from others is not always considered to be a positive situation and can result in discomfort and insensitivity.

Because effective communication is the key to a well-run unit, it is imperative to focus on communication styles and methods and on constantly improving the messages by both senders and receivers.

Some areas of misperceptions resulting from cultural differences include someone's work habits, timeliness, professionalism, integrity, abilities, and level of competency. All these characteristics may be misinterpreted when two members of different cultures do not view the characteristics similarly. One culture may emphasize arriving at work early or even on time, whereas to another culture, this is not that important. Likewise, another culture may place a great deal of emphasis in the family and ensuring that all family members are included in the decision-making process, whereas another may only include males as potential decision makers. Some cultures will not allow male nurses to care for female clients; in other cultures, this is not an issue. Touch is another area of different expectations. In some cultures, only the most necessary touching is done, whereas in others, touching between strangers is not unusual.

Nonverbal communications can sometimes be just as strong as verbal communications, but again, this is an area that can be culturally bound and full of misinterpretations. Personal space, direct eye contact, and body posturing can vary depending on the culture, as can the use of silence. In some cultures, silence is a reflection of what is being said, and it is kept out of respect for the speaker. In other cultures, silence can be a little frustrating.

2. Discuss some of the steps that you, as the manager, need to take to better understand your employees.

Because you are not of the predominately Spanish culture, one of the first things to do is to learn about the employee's culture. Read about the culture; and ask your employees about their culture, their values, their beliefs, their traditions— anything that is important to them as people first and employees second.

Knowing that communication is the key to understanding one another, try to improve on communication techniques. One idea is be to make sure that important information is written down and not trusted to verbal communication—and the informal grapevine. Otherwise, accuracy may become an issue. Another idea is to obtain the trust and understanding of someone of the other culture to help in interpreting your message to the employees and the employees' messages back to you. Watch carefully for the nonverbal responses; many times, people will nod agreement when they really have no notion of what they are agreeing to—or even understand what was said. Finally, listen carefully, and be prepared to rephrase the message that you are sending, especially if someone is nodding agreement but there is a feeling of limited—or even no—comprehension of what is being said or asked.

3. What can you do to help your employees understand your cultural background and communication style?

Part of being an effective manager is first to understand how you communicate as well as how your communication is perceived by others. Communication is affected greatly by perceptions, with both verbal and nonverbal impressions often being influenced by cultural differences. The first rule of order is not to make assumptions about others; ask for clarification of a situation, even when you think you may know the answer. Validate your perceptions.

To help your employees understand you better, you need to know what is are important to you. What are your values, beliefs, and traditions that encompass you as a person? If you are not sure what is important, how can you expect your staff to know? All these aspects are influenced by our environment and background, with regional differences also sometimes becoming significant and illustrating that not all members of a given race or culture act in similar ways. It is well accepted that people from the Mid-Atlantic states of New Jersey and New York have different mannerisms from those who are from Alabama or Mississippi, yet all may be of one race. Some staff members may not have any experience with people from various areas of the country, requiring some awareness training. Likewise, someone moving to Miami from another region of the south may not have had much exposure to people of different cultures and races and would need just as much diversity and awareness education.

Case Scenario 23-2

As the charge nurse in the Emergency Department, you encounter all types of challenging situations. Christopher Wells, a 24-year-old male, is admitted as a trauma victim of a motor vehicle accident. He has extensive injuries, including two broken legs and a punctured lung. After x-ray confirmation, you are calling the operating room to inform the staff of Mr. Wells' pending admission when one of the staff nurses informs you that Mr. Wells' fiancé has just arrived. She is bringing you a copy of a Medical Alert card in his wallet that states he is a Jehovah's Witness and wishes that, in an emergency situation, he refuses all blood and blood products. It is signed by Mr. Wells and by his physician. You find the surgeon who is attempting to obtain a medical history to inform him of your new knowledge.

Case Considerations

1. Define the legal obligations of a medical center to treat a patient who enters through the Emergency Department for care.
2. Describe three options the surgeon has in this scenario and the ramifications of each.
3. Is the surgeon able to perform surgery without administering a blood transfusion? Identify his alternatives to a blood transfusion.
4. Are there legal ramifications if, in an emergency situation, the surgeon knowingly administers blood to a Jehovah's Witness?
5. Are there any blood products that a Jehovah's Witness will accept?
6. How would the care differ if the trauma victim was an 8-year-old child of the Jehovah's Witness faith who required surgery?

Case Analysis

Jehovah's Witnesses are deeply religious people who believe that any blood transfusion is prohibited. They refer to several passages in the Bible to support this belief. Jehovah's Witnesses do accept and actively seek medical and surgical care. The situation becomes more complicated, however, when there is a medical indication for blood—whether whole blood, red blood cells, platelets, or plasma. A Jehovah's Witness will accept the use of heart-lung or dialysis equipment if it is nonblood-prime and their extracorporeal circulation is uninterrupted. Because their understanding of blood products does not so clearly forbid albumin or immune globulins, it is up to the individual Jehovah's Witness to decide whether these materials can be part of a treatment plan, if necessary. All Jehovah's Witnesses accept treatments using colloid or crystalloid replacement fluids. Autologous transfusions, however, are refused.

■ KEY POINTS

1. The critical first step in caring for a person of faith with beliefs that differ from your own is to have knowledge. If you do not know what a specific religion holds as their beliefs, then ask, because some religions, such as Jehovah's Witnesses, have a direct bearing on medical care.
2. Do not assume that just because someone enters the health care system through the Emergency Department that one desires all the medical treatments that can be offered. Consent still needs to be obtained. If the situation is critical the patient is unable to give consent, however, then consent is assumed.
3. If you are unfamiliar with a patient's beliefs and religious convictions, often the patient or family members are glad to educate both you and the entire health care team so that optimal care can be rendered.
4. The hospital chaplain, although perhaps not a member of the patient's particular faith, can be called on for assistance and clarification of religious viewpoints.

Case Scenario 23-3

You are one of two team leaders of a 32-bed medical-oncology unit. Tonight, two other team members, another RN and an unlicensed assistant, are working with you to care for 16 patients. All your patients are fairly stable, except for Mrs. Chen, a 65-year-old woman who immigrated from China with her husband 45 years ago. She has two children, a son and a daughter, who both live in the same neighborhood as their mother. Mrs. Chen understands English, but she speaks the language poorly and prefers to communicate in Chinese.

Mrs. Chen was admitted yesterday to the floor with a metastatic cancer to the pancreas. Her primary cancer was breast cancer, which was treated 6 years ago with surgery and chemotherapy. Her children are taking turns staying at her bedside; they appear to be quite overwhelmed by this hospitalization. It is obvious from her facial gestures and difficulty in moving that Mrs. Chen is in a great deal of pain, but when the RN on your team asks Mrs. Chen about her pain, she just looks at the RN with confusion and states that she is "ok." The son pulls the RN aside and asks why the nurses are not giving his mother pain medication, because she is in obvious pain and discomfort.

When the RN looks over to Mrs. Chen's bedside table at the uneaten meal tray, she notices several brown glass jars containing a variety of liquids and creams, some of them actually smelling rank. The family says that Mrs. Chen believes that she needs the Western doctors and their medicine but still uses traditional Chinese medicine. She has these concoctions made for her by the Chinese herbalist who lives in her city. The nurse also notices that while the room is comfortably warm, Mrs. Chen has on at least five layers of clothing.

Case Considerations

1. Identify several issues that appear in this scenario about Mrs. Chen. Which issue takes priority, and why? How would the other issues rank, and why?
2. Discuss the cultural considerations in caring for Mrs. Chen.
3. Define how you would assess Mrs. Chen's pain more accurately.
4. Are there any issues with Mrs. Chen practicing more traditional Chinese medicine? How would you address this with her physician? Are they harmful?
5. Describe how you would assist Mrs. Chen's son and daughter with their mother's hospitalization. What are the cultural values of family for the traditional Chinese, and how do they affect this hospitalization?
6. What could be some helpful techniques to improve communication between Mrs. Chen and the health care team?
7. Describe several nursing actions that the RN could take to comfort and reassure Mrs. Chen.

Case Analysis

Cultural differences can become barriers when managing patient care if clarification and understanding are not sought early in the relationship. Although Mrs. Chen has been in the United States for many years, she is still not fluent in communicating her needs and desires in English, and she cannot be expected to do so. It is important that we, as caretakers, have realistic expectations of our clients and that these expectations take into account cultural, racial, gender, age, religious, and other differences.

■ KEY POINTS

1. Just because someone has lived for many years in the United States does not automatically give that person competency in the English language. Many immigrants continue to live in

their own ethnic communities, where the native tongue, folkways, and traditions are practiced daily.

2. If there is a language gap, enlist a patient's family or significant others to assist as much as possible in communicating needs.

3. Many cultures do not outwardly express pain, whereas others are quite vocal about not only their pain but also many other emotional issues.

4. Foods are central to many cultures, so allowing native foods, unless they are medically contraindicated, actually may benefit the patient.

5. Some cultures look to the nurse and doctors as people with authority, so they may not question procedures or treatments even when it would be in their best interest to do so.

6. Regardless of the culture, family is always critical to maintaining mental health, particularly during an illness such as Mrs. Chen's. It is always better to work out an arrangement with the family before issues occur and to include the family in the patient's care as much as possible, if for no other reason than to relieve the patient from constant worry.

References

Campinha-Bacote, J. (1994). Cultural competence in psychiatric nursing: A conceptual model. *Nursing Clinics of North America, 29,* 1–8.

Giger, J. N., & Davidhizer, R. E. (1999). *Transcultural nursing.* Baltimore, MD: Mosby.

Leininger, M. (1997). Transcultural nursing research to transform nursing education and practice: 40 years. *Image, 29* (4), 341–347.

Spector, R. (2000). *Cultural diversity in health and illness.* Norwalk, CT: Appleton & Lange.

U.S. Bureau of the Census. (1990).

Suggested Readings

American Association of Colleges of Nursing. (1997). *Statement on diversity and equality of opportunity.* Washington, D.C.: Author.

American Association of Colleges of Nursing. (1998). *Essentials of baccalaureate education for professional nursing practice.* Washington, D.C.: Author.

Andrews, M. M. & Boyle, J. S. (1995). *Transcultural concepts in nursing care.* Philadelphia: J. B. Lippincott.

Burchum, J. L. R. (2002). Cultural competence: An evolutionary perspective. *Nursing Forum, 37* (4), 5–15.

Campinha-Bacote, J., Yahle, T., & Langenkamp, M. (1996). The challenge of cultural diversity for nurse educators. *The Journal of Continuing Education in Nursing, 27* (2), 59–64.

Cox, Jr., T., & Beale, R. L. (2002). *Developing competency to manage diversity.* San Francisco: Berrett-Koehler Publishers.

Geissler, E. M. (1994). *Pocket guide to cultural assessment.* Baltimore, MD: Mosby.

Joint Commission on Accreditation of Healthcare Organizations. (2000). *Comprehensive manual for hospitals: The official handbook.* Oakbrook Terrace, IL: Author.

Hofstede, G. (1997). *Cultures and organizations.* New York: McGraw-Hill.

Long, A. (1997). Nursing: A spiritual perspective. *Nursing Ethics, 4,* 496–510.

Luckman, J. (1999). *Transcultural communication in nursing.* New York: Delmar Publications.

Morrison, T., Conaway, W. A., & Borden, G. A. (1994). *Kiss, bow or shake hands.* Holbkook, MA: Adams Media Corporation.

O'Brien, M. E. (1999). *Spirituality in nursing.* Sudbury, MA: Jones and Bartlett Publishers.

Parsons, L. C. (2002). Transcultural communication: The cornerstone to transcultural care. *SCI Nursing, 19* (4), 160, 162–163.

Peterson, R., Whitman, H., & Smith, J. (1997). A survey of multicultural awareness among hospital and clinic staff. *Journal of Nursing Care Quality, 11* (6), 52–59.

Polifko-Harris, K. (2000). Managing a culturally diverse workforce. In L. M. Simms, S. A. Price, & N. E. Ervin (Eds.), *Professional Practice of Nursing Administration* (pp. 567–581). Albany, NY: Delmar Learning.

Purnell, L. D., & Paulanka, B. J. (1998). *Transcultural health care.* Philadelphia: F. A. Davis.

Stoll, R. (1989). The essence of spirituality. In V. Carson (Ed.), *Spiritual Dimensions of Nursing Practice* (pp. 4–23). Philadelphia: W. B. Saunders.

Taylor, R. (1998). Check our cultural competence. *Nursing Management, 29* (8), 30–32.

Thiederman, S. (1996). Improving communications in a diverse healthcare environment. *Healthcare Financial Management*, November, 72–75.

Walters, C. M. (1999). Professional nursing support for culturally diverse family members of critically ill adults. *Research in Nursing and Health, 22,* 107–117.

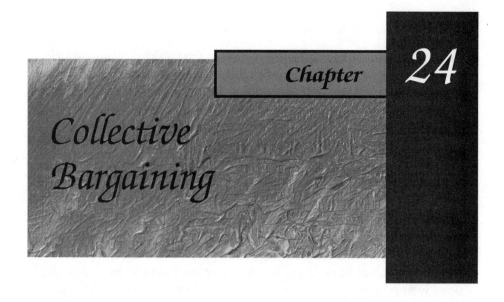

Collective Bargaining

Essential Concepts of Collective Bargaining

Collective bargaining is a legislated right in the United States, but the action itself often invokes strong opinions either for or against the action. Collective bargaining has been part of the fabric of the American workplace since the eighteenth century, when artisans and craftspeople banded together to ensure fair wages. Major legislation protecting the rights of employees was enacted predominantly in the twentieth century. Such legislation includes the National Labor Relations Act of 1935, the Taft-Hartley Act of 1947, and the Landrum-Griffin Act of 1959. The late twentieth century brought two health care–specific acts. First, Executive Order 10988, signed by President Kennedy in 1962, established the right of workers to organize in federal hospitals, but it prevented them from striking. Second, the Taft-Hartley Amendments developed health care–specific rules regarding union activities (Starr, 1982).

Nursing membership in the collective bargaining arena is a relatively new development, with much of the activity spanning perhaps only the last 30 years. Nurses will join a collective bargaining unit for many of the same reasons that others do, with the primary reason being workplace dissatisfaction—especially economic dissatisfaction. The American Nurses Association (ANA) has taken the lead in promoting its representation of professional nurses in the workplace, and in 1949, the ANA registered as a bargaining agent for nurses that acts through the individual state nurses associations (Tazbir, 2003). It is estimated that more than half the nurses who are members of unions are represented by these state organizations.

Models of Collective Action

- Workplace advocacy is a type of collective action activity that encompasses nurses who strive to alter policies, procedures, or methods to improve an outcome.
- Formal collective bargaining is often accomplished within organizations where staffing levels are considered to be unsafe, morale poor, communication between management and staff inadequate, and wages low.
- Other issues that may encourage a union environment include real or perceived discrimination and favoritism among staff. A union environment encourages managers to treat everyone equally, including fair performance evaluations.
- If disputes occur in the work setting between the manager and the employee, several options can be found in a unionized setting, including grievance, mediation, and arbitration procedures to ensure a fair outcome.

The American Nurses Association and Collective Bargaining

- The ANA is the professional organization for the representation of registered nurses (RNs) in the United States. It has been recognized by the National Labor Relations Board as a collective bargaining unit since 1949.
- Because the ANA represents all nurses, conflict sometimes occurs between those nurses who consider joining a union unprofessional and those who rely on the influence of the ANA to provide a better work environment.
- A portion of the ANA is devoted to the work of its union arm, but the ANA also has significant interest in the welfare and setting of standards for nurses and their patients. Additionally, the ANA lobbies Congress and other influential politicians about those issues affecting nurses, the delivery of effective health care, and the promotion of safe, quality nursing care.

Professionalism and Unionization

- Nurses have long viewed themselves as professionals, yet some argue that professionals do not organize into unions.
- Supervisors or managers are not admitted into a union. Depending on the institutional definition of a staff nurse, some may be considered inappropriate for union admission unless their job description clearly states that they are employees, not supervisors of other nursing employees.
- Certain physicians are also joining unions in an effort to halt their loss of autonomy and decreasing wages while maintaining their autonomy of practice.

Pros and Cons of Collective Bargaining

- When a health care setting is threatened with union activity by one or more of its employee groups, management, understandably, becomes apprehensive and anxious. Many nurses believe that a union on-site will result in pay raises and lower staffing ratios, but other issues need to be considered as well. Some of these issues include conforming to the vote of the group members, the loss of individuality, and an organization that professionals do not join.

CASE SCENARIOS

Guided Case Scenario 24-1

The RN vacancy rate has been consistently more than 15% for the last 3 years at the hospital where you are one of five medical-surgical nurse managers. Because of this high vacancy rate, many agency nurses are working, particularly during the off-shifts. You hear that the hospital nurses are frustrated with the staffing patterns, which often places the nurses in uncomfortable situations because of the lack of professional staff.

Because you are having an evening staff meeting, you come in late today and find several of your staff RNs talking in the hallway. When you approach, they become quiet. You are curious about their behavior, so the first person you look for is your assistant manager. He informs you that because of the high vacancy rate and the resulting poor staffing patterns, the Vice President of Nursing has just sent out a new policy entitled "Mandatory Overtime for

Registered Nurse Staff." Your assistant says that he is worried, because according to the informal grapevine in the hospital, a union
representative has been contacted and there is now significant interest in bringing in a union specifically for the nurses.

Case Considerations

1. What are some of the reasons why nurses would, or would
   not, join a union? What are some of the motivating factors to
   join a union? Describe the optimal environment in which
   union activity may be developed. What would be the most
   significant influence on your decision?
2. Describe the rights that an employee has in participating in
   union organization.
3. Do you believe that you, as a manager, have responsibilities to
   your staff as they explore the possibility of collective bargaining?
4. Identify the main steps in the organization of a collective
   bargaining unit.

Case Analysis

1. What are some of the reasons why nurses would, or would
   not, join a union? What are some of the motivating factors to
   join a union? Describe the optimal environment in which
   union activity may be developed. What would be the most
   significant influence on your decision?

   Many of the same issues often motivate RNs, and these
   issues become even more obvious in times of nursing shortages. Often, RNs turn to collective bargaining agents when
   they feel that they are no longer heard or understood by the
   management of their institution. The nurses may have
   complaints about unsafe staffing, poor pay, unsafe work conditions, job insecurity, and poor quality of care. They often feel
   that the nurse administrators do not effectively communicate
   with them, neither hearing their issues nor attempting to
   understand them. Nurses may also want a union because they
   feel that favoritism or inequality exists in some facet of the
   workplace and that a union will end the discrimination.

   On the other hand, many nurses do not feel it is professional
   to join a union, and they may have great difficulty even with
   the dual purpose of the ANA, which on the one hand
   represents all RNs and on the other is the largest collective
   bargaining agent for professional nurses. Other issues that

nurses may have that weigh against joining a union include the need to not be part of a system that everyone else is a part of, that it is a "blue-collar mentality," and that the hospital may somehow retaliate if they are union members. To make an informed decision, it is imperative that one examines their own values and belief sets about professional nursing before participating in any collective bargaining activities.

2. Describe the rights that an employee has in participating in union organization.

Under the National Labor Relations Act of 1935, employees have the right to participate in union organizing. Also known as the Wagner Act, this legislation established the rights of the employees to organize and to bargain collectively, initially covered the health care industry, and has been amended three times (Starr, 1982). Essentially, every private employee has the right to organize.

Those nurses participating in unionization need to be cautious and follow labor law carefully while working with a collective bargaining agent. Meeting times should not interfere with direct patient care activities unless adequate coverage exists. It is best that organizing meetings occur around shift change and that everyone, including management, knows when they are occurring. An employee cannot be fired simply for participating in an organizing union unless some inappropriate behavior, such as leaving patients without necessary coverage to attend meetings also occurs.

3. Do you believe that you, as a manager, have responsibilities to your staff as they explore the possibility of collective bargaining?

Managers, historically, are not part of the collective bargaining agreements, because only the staff are participants in the union. It is especially critical that if a manager hears about collective bargaining activity, he or she becomes well versed in the reasons that have driven the employees to this point. The more informed that management is about the causative factors and the issues of the employees, the less cantankerous the situation may become during bargaining and developing the contract between union members and representatives of management.

The manager has a specific role to play when a union is in its beginning stages. First, managers should know that they are representing the hospital and the hospital administration during the union organization, so they should be cautious as to their participation levels with their staff. Both management and employees have clear-cut responsibilities and rights, and it is imperative that managers not overstep their boundaries Second, managers should stay within their delegated duties, regardless of what others may try to force them to do. The law does cover employees' rights. Third, while the manager cannot actively attempt to prohibit employees from meeting, or voting, the management staff can attempt to help the employees to understand the ramifications of joining a union and what having a union will mean to the daily operations of the hospital, including patient care outcomes. Generally, wages will go up within a union shop, but there may be other activities that will no longer be funded. The most important thing to remember as a manager is to actively listen to the employees' issues and concerns.

4. Identify the main steps in the organization of a collective bargaining unit.

Regardless of the setting, there are consistent steps to follow when an organization is in the union development phase. The first step is to ascertain who is interested in a union developing at the institution. To hold an election for collective bargaining to occur, the National Labor Relations Board requires that at least 30% of the total number of potential enrollees show interest via a card vote. An institution is then required to hold an election if there is at least a 30% interest shown. All lines of communication should be kept open between managers, staff, and the collective bargaining agent. In addition, the health care industry has several differences compared to other industries, such as federal facilities not being allowed to strike. Once the vote is taken and there is a move to the formal recognition of the unit, a contract is negotiated. The primary areas of contract negotiation are typically wages, grievances, and workplace rules and discipline.

Case Scenario 24-2

As a new BSN graduate, you have the option of working at either of the two large hospital systems in the city where you live. Both hospital systems offer many of the same clinical opportunities, and both have wonderful preceptor programs. The primary difference is that one has a collective bargaining unit for their RNs and the other one does not. The health care system with the collective bargaining unit has slightly higher wages and some other additional benefits compared to the facility without collective bargaining. You are offered jobs with both health care systems.

Case Considerations

1. Deciding which health care system to take a job in is a major decision. Should the notion of one health care system having a collective bargaining unit for its RNs be a consideration for you? Why, or why not?
2. What are the ramifications of working in a health care environment that maintains a collective bargaining unit for its RNs?
3. What are some of the potentially favorable outcomes from working in a health care environment that maintains a collective bargaining unit for its RNs?
4. Describe your thought processes about making a decision about in which facility to begin employment. What is the leading factor for you in this decision?
5. Which facility will you choose to work in, and what can you reasonably expect as far as the work environment?

Case Analysis

Whether one is an experienced nurse or someone just out of school, there are many factors to consider when taking a new position at a new facility. Factors such as pay, schedules, work environment, and patient assignments are all critical, but it is also important to consider additional issues when there is an active collective bargaining unit specifically for RNs.

■ KEY POINTS

1. When there is a collective bargaining unit at a health care facility, the union does not always require that everyone in a particular category to join to receive the benefits. One of the areas to check carefully are the requirements for membership and whether payment of dues is required regardless of membership status.
2. The ANA has a dual purpose: It is the official organization for RNs, and at the same time, it is a collective bargaining agent.
3. Labor relation legislation often is written to describe the relationships between the employers and the union that represents the employees.

4. There are numerous motivating factors to join a union, just as there are many reasons not to join a collective bargaining unit. Joining a union is often a personal decision, depending on one's values and expectations of the workplace as well as the employer.

5. Employees are often more motivated to join a collective bargaining unit when there is generalized unhappiness regarding workplace conditions, whether that unhappiness is driven by money, patients, or assignments.

References

Starr, P. (1982). *The social transformation of American medicine.* New York: Basic Books.

Tazbir, J. (2003). Collective bargaining. In P. Kelly-Heidenthal (Ed.), *Nursing leadership and management.* Clifton Park, NY: Delmar Learning.

Suggested Readings

Aiken, T. D. (1994). *Legal, ethical, and political issues in nursing.* Philadelphia: F. A. Davis.

Hart, C. (1998). The state of the unions. *Nursing Times, 94* (15), 36–37.

Lundy, M. C. (1997). How nurses can organize for the purposes of collective bargaining. *Revolution—The Journal of Nurse Empowerment, 7* (4), 38.

Marquis, B. L., & Huston, C. J. (2000). *Leadership roles and management functions* (3rd ed.). Philadelphia: J. B. Lippincott.

Melville, E. (1995). The history of industrial action in nursing. *Professional Nurse, 11* (2), 84–86.

Phan, C. (1999). Physician unionization: The impact on the medical profession. *Journal of Legal Medicine, 20* (1), 114–140.

Porter-O'Grady, T. (2001). Collective bargaining: The union as partner. *Nursing Management, 32* (6, pt. 1), 3–32.

Rabben, T. (1991). Is unionization compatible with professionalism? *Industrial and Labor Relations Review, 45* (1), 97–110.

Rowland, H. S., & Rowland, B. L. (1997). *Nursing administration handbook* (4th ed.). Gaithersburg, MD: Aspen Publishers.

Seltzer, T. M. (2001). Collective bargaining: A wake-up call-part 2. *Nursing Management, 32* (4), 35–37, 48.

Simms, L. M., Price, S. A., & Ervin, N. E. (2000). *Professional practice of nursing administration* (3rd ed.). Clifton Park, NY: Delmar Learning.

Stearley, H. (1995). The rise and fall of nursing unions. *Revolution—The Journal of Nurse Empowerment, 5* (2), 56–59.

The role of collective bargaining and unions in advancing the profession of nursing. (1998). *Nursing Trends & Issues, 3* (2), 1–8.

UNIT

Preparation for Entry-Level Nursing Practice

VII

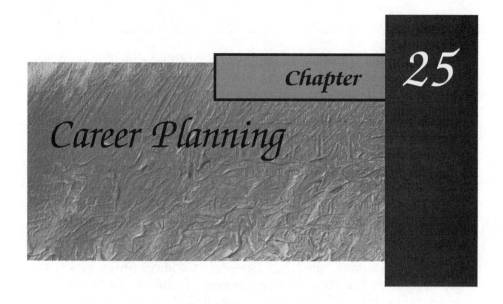

Chapter 25

Career Planning

Essential Concepts of Career Planning

Graduation is a time to begin a new career or take on additional responsibilities in a current job. Careers as a registered nurse (RN) are plentiful, with multiple opportunities in a variety of roles and positions. Today, obtaining a job is easier for an RN than it has been in a long time, but some points still need to be kept in mind during the search process to ensure that the position taken is the right decision.

The most important step before starting is to do a self-assessment. Identify those areas in which you excel and those in which you need to improve, and identify situations that are exciting and that are mundane. This will assist you in seeking the correctly paced professional environment.

There are many factors to consider when job hunting. Sometimes, an opportunity just presents itself, such as an offer made by a manager who has seen the work of a potential employee during a clinical rotation. However, that situation is more the exception than the rule; therefore, you need to begin with the first step of preparing for the search. With so many job openings even in one city, it is imperative that the applicant makes a listing, in ranking order, of those things that are important, such as schedule, pay, education and training, promotional opportunities, and distance from home before sending out resumes to all available institutions. Once an interview is obtained, it is helpful to research the institution and make sure there will be a good fit—especially when it comes to the mission, values, and expectations of employees. Talking with current employees (other than the recruiter) will often yield honest answers to these questions, and these answers should be considered in the overall decision-making process of interviewing.

The Successful Job Search

- The most important—and the first—step in a successful job search is preparation. You should know the area of clinical practice in which you excel (did you have a great clinical experience on a certain unit?) or in which you would like more experience. As a new graduate, you may not be able to secure your first choice, with many facilities requiring a certain amount of experience other than clinical experience in school.
- Before securing interviews, perform a thorough self-assessment.
- When reviewing options for your first position, you may want to ask a trusted colleague for insight regarding your strengths and weaknesses. If you enjoy ambiguity and reacting at the last minute, a position in the Emergency Department may be your first choice.
- Even when you take you first position, it is not too early to begin career planning. If you are an experienced RN, your BSN may open up new opportunities for you to investigate and expand the horizons of your career past the clinical area. Many management positions, for example, require the minimum of a BSN.
- One can use several resources in the job search. The first would be direct experience. Where did you do a clinical that was both satisfying and challenging? The employment bulletin boards in the Human Resources Department generally lists all the open positions within an institution.
- Newspapers and trade journals are a common place to locate job openings. The ads may not be indicative of all the openings a facility has, however, or the ad may be focused only on a hard-to-fill position.
- Electronic media, such as websites and job boards with multiple job opportunities, are becoming increasingly popular, offering a job applicant the ability to search a variety of employers at a glance.

- Another important piece to the job search is networking. Who works at an institution in which you are interested? They may know of a job opportunity even before it is advertised, or they may be able to act as your reference. Keep in mind that not all jobs are advertised, and one of the only ways one can find out about some jobs is through word-of-mouth.

Developing a Resume

- Most resumes contain certain elements: the heading, career objective, professional experience, formal education, and possibly, awards, honors, and references (Table 25-1).
- The purpose of a resume is to get the attention of a potential employer so that at least an initial interview occurs. Using action verbs can help (Table 25-2).
- There are two primary types of resumes. The chronological resume lists jobs in reverse chronological order. The functional resume groups skills and abilities together rather than have specific listing for jobs.
- A cover letter should always accompany a resume. The cover letter is a way of introducing yourself by presenting the highlights of your resume.

Dressing for the Interview

- Business attire is the accepted dress for an interview. If you are interviewing for a staff nurse position, you do not need to show up for the interview in a three-piece suit, but one should also not show up in jeans and sandals. Makeup, perfume, and jewelry should be kept at a minimum.

Interview Questions

- Regardless of your experience in interviewing, it is always helpful to practice answering potential questions before the interview so that you can discover which may be difficult to answer. One question that most prospective employers ask—and that potential employees always are stumped on—is the proverbial "What are your strengths and weaknesses?" By role playing with possible questions and answers, you can evaluate your responses before you have to do it in front of a prospective employer. It also gives you an opportunity to think of possible situations that you have handled well and how you have reacted (or would react) in certain environments. You can never be too prepared for an interview.

Table 25-1   Elements of a Resume

Identifying information/ heading	Include your name, address, telephone number, and e-mail address. If you are moving after school, be sure to include a permanent address.
Career objective	Specify your employment target to help recruiters quickly identify your purpose in applying.
Employment data/ professional experience	Include name of employer, location of employer, dates employed, and job title(s). If you are developing a chronological resume, write about specific job responsibilities, job skills, and any accomplishments while you were employed at each agency or facility. If you are writing a functional resume, include only the name and address of the employer, dates employed, and job title(s). Include relevant clinical experiences, specialty classes, preceptorships, externships, or research projects.
	Keep in mind that prospective employers are interested in your ability to work well with the public and other employees, your positive communication skills, and your ability to maintain a strong work ethic.
Military experience	Include rank, service, assignment, dates, and significant experiences.
Formal education and specialized training	Note where you attended school, the school's address, the degree you received (e.g., BSN), the date you completed your studies, and any special achievements, such as grade point average (especially if it was 3.0 or better), any leadership positions held, any membership in student or professional organizations, and any specialized training.
Professional organizations and memberships	Identify memberships and any offices held.
Awards and honors (optional)	If you are a new graduate without a significant work history, you could include high school and college honors and awards.
References	The statement "References available upon request" can be placed on the last line of a resume. You can either provide a listing of references on the application or bring a separate reference list to a job interview. Include at least three professional references, with names, titles, addresses, and phone numbers—but only after receiving permission from these persons to use them as references. Do not use family, friends, or neighbors as references. Notify your references when you interview to let them know they may be contacted.

Table 25-2   List of Action Verbs for a Resume

accomplished	developed	listed	reduced
achieved	directed	maintained	reengineered
administered	earned	managed	reinforced
analyzed	eliminated	mastered	reorganized
approved	established	motivated	revamped
built	evaluated	negotiated	revised
communicated	expanded	operated	simplified
completed	explored	organized	solved
conceived	generated	oversaw	streamlined
conducted	identified	performed	supervised
coordinated	increased	planned	taught
created	initiated	proposed	terminated
delivered	innovated	provided	trained
demonstrated	instituted	purchased	transformed
designed	launched	redesigned	utilized

- At the interview, do not forget to ask questions about the orientation process and the preceptorship. How long does it last? Who will be the preceptors? How will the evaluation process occur, and how often? When is it determined that a new employee is ready to come off orientation? Can staffing issues dictate a quick end to orientation?
- Keep in mind that you are interviewing the prospective employer as well as being interviewed as a prospective employee. You need to come prepared to ask them pertinent questions about issues that you deem to be important, such as schedule flexibility, pay raises and differentials, education and training, and opportunities to move up within the organization.

CASE SCENARIOS

Guided Case Scenario 25-1

Amy, a new graduate, has secured an interview for a staff nurse position in the neonatal intensive care unit (NICU) at the Children's Hospital. Most new RNs are not granted interviews until they have had at least a year of experience. The nurse manager has seen Amy work during the last year as a nurse's aide, however, and believes that she has great potential as an RN.

Case Considerations

1. Identify some of Amy's personal characteristics that she would more than likely need to have to be successful in the intensive care environment. How critical is it for her to perform a self-assessment before accepting the interview, especially considering that she has worked in the NICU for a year as a nurse's aide? Is this past employment a guarantee of success as an RN?
2. Because Amy is already an employee of the institution, what questions should she ask her manager?
3. Discuss some of the ways that Amy can prepare for her interview.
4. Identify several pros and cons to taking a new position in a unit where Amy is already an employee.

Case Analysis

1. Identify some of Amy's personal characteristics she would more than likely need to have to be successful in the intensive care environment. How critical is it for her to perform a self-assessment prior to accepting the interview, especially considering that she has worked in the NICU for a year as a nurse's aide? Is this past employment a guarantee of success as an RN?

   Amy's situation is not all that unusual; in fact, she is fortunate that her employer thinks enough of her abilities to invite her for an interview as an RN. The role of nurse's aide is very different from the role of the RN, however, so it is crucial that Amy reflect and do a self-assessment before the interview.

   Working in the intensive care setting takes a certain type of personality, and not everyone who wants to work in this environment has the ability to succeed. One may have the knowledge required by the setting, but there also needs to be a personality "fit." Someone who likes providing in-depth patient care, can make decisions quickly and with frequency, prefers independence, and is assertive generally does well in the fast-paced critical care environment. Likewise, not everyone can succeed in the medical-surgical care, psychiatric care, obstetrical care, or home health specialties, so it is imperative to know your own personality before taking a position in any area of nursing.

2. Because Amy is already an employee of the institution, what questions should she ask her manager?

Just because Amy is already an employee does not automatically guarantee her a position, especially since she is interviewing for a different role. Amy should come prepared to the interview with questions of her own. By having her own set of questions, she is showing the manager that she is organized and has carefully thought about the role for which she is interviewing.

Of course, Amy should ask questions about the expectations of the position. What are the responsibilities? What are the hours? What are the benefits and pay schedule? Amy also needs to go further with her questioning for several reasons. Not only is she seeking information and clarification of the role and responsibilities, but sometimes, when an employee switches roles within the same department, many issues are not well thought out ahead of time. This leaves the employee frustrated and often not working at his or her optimal level.

Amy should ask specific questions about her orientation. How long will it be? Who will be her preceptor? Are there classes for her to attend? What is the proposed schedule? What is her pay?

An area that many potential employees forget about is the evaluative component of a new job. How often can Amy expect formal feedback and evaluation of her progress in her new role as an RN? What are the ramifications of lack of progress? What type of assistance will she receive if needed?

3. Discuss some of the ways that Amy can prepare for her interview.

Amy can prepare for her interview in a variety of ways, but the most important is to anticipate the questions that she will be asked. Amy also needs to determine the questions that she will want to ask the manager. Amy should be ready to answer the usual questions. Why do you want to work in this unit? What skills do you bring to the position? What are your strengths and weaknesses? Why do you want to work in the intensive care setting? What personal characteristics would make you successful in the intensive care setting? Tell me about a success that you have had and a failure you have had. What did you learn from both situations? Do you anticipate any problems with leaving your role as a nurse's aide and transitioning to the RN role? Why should we hire you?

4. Identify several pros and cons to taking a new position in a unit where Amy is already an employee.

Amy needs to consider several things if she is offered the position of RN in the NICU where she has been employed as a nurse's aide for the past year. Most important, she is currently viewed by the staff as a subordinate: She is a nurse's aide and a nursing student. It may be difficult for her to transition to the role of professional RN, to take on an equal role to that of the staff. The situation may go one of two ways: Amy may have difficulty in gaining the confidence of the staff because of her previous role as a nurse's aide, or they may take her under their guidance, wanting her to succeed.

Amy also needs to be prepared for the role change and for the expectations that the role change will bring. There are many positive aspects to obtaining a promotion in the same department, such as familiarity of staff, procedures, location of supplies, and other health care team members. On the other hand, there are certain cons that Amy needs to be cognizant of if she accepts this new role, including the anticipation of role change, confidence of the staff, higher expectations of others (because she does have the knowledge), and a potentially shortened orientation timeframe (again because of her familiarity with the environment). Whenever someone accepts a promotion or begins a new role in the same department, the expectations of both the employee and the employer need to be clearly delineated before the new position begins so that the employee and the department receive the maximum benefit.

Case Scenario 25-2

Rebecca will be graduating from an accelerated BSN program at the end of the summer semester, and she needs to prepare for the interviewing process regarding a position in the local hospital. Rebecca is not the typical college student. She is 50 years old, has two teenage children, and had an extremely successful career in real estate sales when she decided to change careers and go into the nursing field.

Case Considerations

1. As Rebecca prepares her resume, how should she discuss her past employment history? Is it important? What key points should be made on her resume?

2. Identify at least six transferable skills from Rebecca's real estate career to her new career as an RN. Are there any similarities between her previous career and her new career?
3. What type of questions can Rebecca anticipate during the interviewing process?
4. Describe several questions that a prospective employer may—but from the legal perspective really should not—ask Rebecca.
5. What can Rebecca predict as some of the areas of concern that a prospective employer may have in hiring her? What are some of the strengths that Rebecca would bring to a nursing unit?

Case Analysis

One of the attractions of the nursing profession is that one can enter at almost any point in their working life and become successful in a variety of settings. However, it is wise to anticipate some of the potential issues that a prospective employer may have in hiring an older, work-experienced employee—however unfounded those issues may be.

■ KEY POINTS

1. It is imperative that Rebecca spend some time in developing her resume and her interviewing techniques. It has been a long time since she has looked for employment, and some of her interviewing skills may need refining.
2. The resume is the key to getting an interview, so it may be beneficial to have another professional review the resume before sending it to a prospective employer.
3. A cover letter is critical to introducing a candidate to a prospective employer.
4. It is advantageous to practice for an upcoming interview with a colleague or a friend, especially when interviewing skills may need polishing.
5. Certain questions cannot be asked of an employee because of Equal Employment Opportunity and Affirmative Action rules. Make sure that the candidate is well aware of these questions, and how to indirectly answer them.
6. Potential questions should be anticipated, and practice answers should be derived before the interview itself.

Case Scenario 25-3

Ron is a retired naval captain who is enrolled in the second-degree program, an accelerated BSN program. He has done phenomenally well in nursing school, with high test averages and successful clinical rotations in the area hospitals and health care systems. Ron is in his final semester and wishes to look for employment as an RN in the specialty that he really enjoys: obstetrics. There are openings in the mother-baby unit at the local hospital, and they have a preceptorship for new graduates. However, when Ron calls for an interview, they are hesitant, saying that they already have many applicants who are female and would like to give preference to them first. Ron turns to you, an experienced nurse manager, for assistance.

Case Considerations

1. Is there an issue here? If so, define it. Should there be an issue?
2. Analyze some of the barriers that men in nursing sometimes need to overcome in a predominately female profession.
3. Discuss how you, as the manager, could advise Ron as he attempts to secure an interview for an obstetrical staff nurse position.
4. When Ron obtains the interview, what could be some areas of strength that he could make sure to bring into the conversation? Identify those areas that he may not want to volunteer during the interview.
5. Should male staff nurses work in the specialty area of mother-baby care? What are some of the pros and cons, and how would you advise Ron?
6. As a retired naval officer, Ron brings a wealth of experience to his new profession. Identify some of those skills and experiences that would be helpful for Ron to mention during his interview process.
7. Do you foresee any potential difficulties that Ron may encounter in his first role as an RN?

Case Analysis

Nursing is currently more than 94% female, so that the males who do work as RNs often have to overcome some boundaries about which their female counterparts may not have had to worry. On the other hand, it is not always a negative to be a male, because there will always be advantages to being a minority male in a predominately female profession.

■ *KEY POINTS*

1. As the nursing shortage continues, there will be many more second-career students entering the nursing profession.
2. Most military branches offer special educational incentives to return to the workplace once someone retires.
3. Many second-career students have skills that are highly transferable to future nursing positions. It is necessary to have already thought of these skills before to the interview process, because a prospective employer may not know the previous career skills well or which of its skills can be applied to nursing.
4. Prejudice often exists for male nurses, particularly in the field of obstetrics. This may be a result of both staff and patient perceptions.
5. Someone in Ron's position needs to be able to communicate effectively his strengths and applicable skills, especially because he is having difficulty in securing an interview. It may be helpful to have a trusted colleague call the recruiter and speak to his qualities.
6. Ron should seek out a mentor, preferably another male, who may be able to assist him in his new career path.

Suggested Readings

Bozell, J. (1999). *Anatomy of a job search—A nurse's guide to finding and landing the job you want.* Philadelphia: Springhouse.

Hadley, J., & Sheldon, B. (1995). *The smart woman's guide to networking.* Philadelphia: Chelsea House Publishers.

Hauter, J. (1997). *The smart woman's guide to career success.* Philadelphia: Chelsea House Publishers.

Kennedy, J. L. (1999). *Resumes for dummies.* Foster City, CA: IDG Books Worldwide.

Lore, N. (1998). *The pathfinder.* New York: Simon & Schuster.

Simms, L. M., Price, S. A. & Ervin, N. E. (2000). *Professional practice of nursing administration* (3rd ed.). Clifton Park, NY: Delmar Learning.

Smith, R. (1999). *Electronic resumes and online networking.* Franklin Lakes, NJ: Career Press.

Welton, R. H., & Morton, P. G. (1995). Strategies for writing an effective resume. *Critical Care Nurse,* June, 118–126.

Index